Nursing history and the politics of welfare

Nursing history has become a robust and reflective area of scholarship, which recognizes the inescapable social, political, economic and cultural factors influencing the profession. *Nursing History and the Politics of Welfare* highlights the significant contribution that researching nursing history has to make in setting a new intellectual and political agenda for nurses.

Reflecting the international scale of current research, eighteen contributors look at nursing from different perspectives, as it has developed under different regimes and ideologies and at different points in time in America, Australia, Britain, Germany, India, the Philippines and South Africa. They examine the ways in which the nursing workforce is segmented and stratified along race, class and gender lines and how differences of culture undermine attempts to theorize nursing and health care in universal terms. Comparing the problems and potential of the 'equal' rights and 'difference' approaches, they propose strategies for achieving greater recognition for nursing, to bring it into line with other related, yet male-dominated professions within the health care arena.

Anne Marie Rafferty is Director of the Centre for Policy in Nursing Research, London School of Hygiene and Tropical Medicine. **Jane Robinson** is Professor and Head of the Department of Nursing and Midwifery Studies, University of Nottingham. **Ruth Elkan** is Research Fellow, Department of Nursing and Midwifery Studies, University of Nottingham.

✳ DATE LABEL OVER PAGE ✳

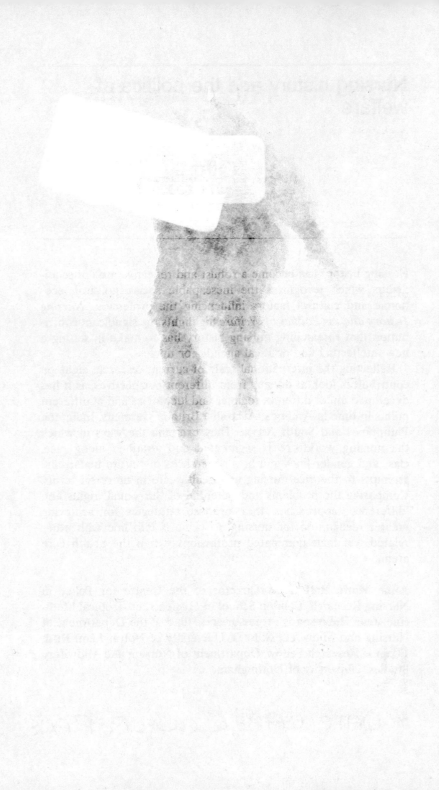

Nursing history and the politics of welfare

Edited by Anne Marie Rafferty,
Jane Robinson and Ruth Elkan

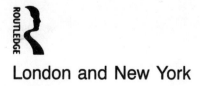

London and New York

First published 1997
by Routledge
11 New Fetter Lane, London EC4P 4EE

Simultaneously published in the USA and Canada
by Routledge
29 West 35th Street, New York, NY 10001

© 1997 Selection and editorial matter, Anne Marie Rafferty, Jane
Robinson and Ruth Elkan; individual chapters, the contributors.

Phototypeset in Times by Intype London Ltd

Printed and bound in Great Britain by
Mackays of Chatham PLC, Chatham, Kent

British Library Cataloguing in Publication Data
A catalogue record for this book is available from the British Library

Library of Congress Cataloging in Publication Data
Nursing history and the politics of welfare/edited by Anne Marie
    Rafferty, Jane Robinson, and Ruth Elkan.
        p. cm.
    Includes bibliographical references and index.
    1. Nursing–History. 2. Public welfare–History. I. Rafferty,
Anne Marie. II. Robinson, Jane, 1935– . III. Elkan, Ruth,
1954– .
    [DNLM: 1. History of Nursing. 2. Politics. WY 11.1 N9739
    1996]
RT31.N864 1996
610.73'09—dc20
DNLM/DLC
for Library of Congress   96–19933
                                                                  CIP

ISBN 0–415–13835–3 (hbk)
ISBN 0–415–13836–1 (pbk)

Contents

Tables

Contributors

Sarah Elise Abrams has extensive experience in public policy analysis in state government and higher education and is continuing to study the impact of Rockefeller Foundation activities in nursing in the USA. She is currently an assistant professor in the College of Nursing, East Tennessee State University.

Ellen D. Baer is director of the nursing doctoral programme and Visiting Professor of Nursing at New York University and Professor Emeritus of Nursing at the University of Pennsylvania. Her PhD is in the history of nursing and her research and writing on that subject have won many major awards. Recently she entered the field of political journalism, authoring or co-authoring articles in major American newspapers on nursing and health care.

Geertje Boschma studied nursing, philosophy and history of nursing, and worked as a psychiatric mental health nurse in the Netherlands and the USA. She obtained a master's degree in mental health nursing from the University of Pennsylvania. She is currently preparing a PhD thesis on the history of Dutch mental health nursing 1820–1920 at the same university and has contributed to the International Council of Nurses Centennial project.

Barbara Brush is an Assistant Professor in the Department of Nursing, Temple University, Philadelphia. She completed her doctoral degree at the University of Pennsylvania as well as a postdoctoral fellowship at the Center for the Study of the History of Nursing. Her research in history and policy, particularly around issues of the nursing workforce, immigration, workforce stratification, and nurse/hospital relations has been the subject of numerous articles and papers as well as a forthcoming co-authored monograph, to be published by Blackwell Science. She will continue her research at Boston College, Chesnut Hill, Massachusetts.

Angela Cushing undertook a bachelor of arts (hons) degree at Monash University, Victoria, Australia, majoring in history. This degree stimulated further study in history which culminated in a PhD in 1989. Subsequently she developed a professional commitment to the history of nursing, oral history and qualitative research. Currently she is the co-ordinator of postgraduate studies in the School of Nursing at Queensland University of Technology and co-ordinator of the Qualitative Research Unit in the Master of Nursing, Graduate Diploma and Bachelor of Nursing (Hons) Programme.

Harriet Deacon is currently a post-doctoral research fellow at Queen's College, Oxford, researching the social history of medicine in the Cape Colony. She did her PhD at the University of Cambridge, on the history of the medical institutions on Robben Island, South Africa, 1846–1910. Her undergraduate degree was from the University of Cape Town.

Ruth Elkan is research fellow in the Department of Nursing and Midwifery Studies at the University of Nottingham. She has researched and written on nursing education, management and research policy.

Rosemary Fitzgerald is Senior Lecturer in the School of Education, Politics and Social Science, South Bank University, London. She has also taught at Oxford University and universities in the USA and Canada. She has carried out research on gender and health service delivery in rural North India and is currently researching the history of medical missions, women and health care in colonial India.

Judith Godden is a historian, Senior Lecturer and Head of the Department of Behavioural and Social Sciences in Nursing at the University of Sydney. She has published widely in the areas of social welfare and nursing history. Her main research and teaching interest is to explore the development of modern nursing in the context of broader social trends and issues.

Lesley Hall is Senior Assistant Archivist, Contemporary Medical Archives Centre, Wellcome Institute for the History of Medicine. Besides being a professional archivist, she has a PhD from the University of London in the history of medicine and has published *Hidden Anxieties: Male Sexuality 1900–1950*, and (with Roy Porter) *The Facts of Life: the Creation of Sexual Knowledge in Britain 1650–1950*, among other titles.

Shula Marks was formerly Director of the Institute of Commonwealth Studies, London and is now Professor of Southern African History at the School of Oriental and African Studies. She has written extensively on South African history. Her most recent book is *Divided Sisterhood: Race, Class and Gender in the South African Nursing Profession* (Macmillan and Wits University Press, 1994). She is currently continuing her research into health care with a book to be entitled *Mothers, Miners and Maniacs: Essays in the Social History of Medicine in South Africa*.

Jennifer Maxwell is completing an ESRC-funded PhD dissertation on the early development of health visiting. She is a qualified nurse, midwife and health visitor and has recently worked as a temporary lecturer in the Department of Nursing and Midwifery Studies at the University of Nottingham. She has also been employed as a local co-ordinator for the Nottinghamshire/ Lincolnshire area of the Trent Health Authority focus for the promotion of research in primary health care.

Barbara Mortimer is English but has lived in Scotland since 1982. A Lecturer in Nursing at Queen Margaret College, Edinburgh, she is also currently a part-time PhD student with the Department of Economic and Social History in the University of Edinburgh, where her research is concerned with clarifying the role of nurses in that city in the early nineteenth century. Her study is supported by a research training fellowship awarded by the National Board for Nursing, Midwifery and Health Visiting for Scotland.

Tom Olson is an Assistant Professor in the School of Nursing at the University of Hawaii-Manoa. His previous publications focus on the organization of general nursing in the USA and the conceptualization of psychiatric nursing. He is currently completing a study of the evolution of concepts and practises related to mental health and illness in early-twentieth-century Hawaii.

Anne Marie Rafferty is Director of the Centre for Policy in Nursing Research at the London School of Hygiene and Tropical Medicine. She has written on the social history of nursing, the politics of nursing knowledge and is co-editing a volume in the history of midwifery.

Jane Robinson is Professor and Head of the Department of Nursing and Midwifery Studies at the University of Nottingham. She has written on the history of health visiting, NHS reforms, nursing policy, nursing management and the theory and practice of health needs assessment. She is Temporary Adviser and consultant to the World Health Organization on a range of nursing policy issues.

Hilde Steppe is a registered nurse, living in Frankfurt/Main, Germany. She qualified in the 1960s and now has further qualifications in intensive-care nursing and nursing management and an MA in education (minor in history). She is currently the leader of the nursing department in the State of Hessen's Ministry of Environment, Energy, Youth, Family and Health. Her special areas of research are: history of nursing; nursing as a woman's profession; nursing in Nazi Germany; and nursing and society.

Glenda Strachan lectures in labour history and industrial relations at the University of Newcastle, Australia. Her research has covered the changes to the occupation of nursing and the development and role of nursing associations in Australia. *Labour of Love: the History of the Nurses' Association in Queensland*, based on her PhD thesis, was published in 1996. She has published a number of articles on nursing and other aspects of women's work, both historical and contemporary.

Acknowledgements

This volume started life as a series of papers delivered at the first 'Nursing History and the Politics of Welfare' conference organized by the Department of Nursing and Midwifery Studies at the University of Nottingham in 1993. Sarah Smith's organizational genius contributed greatly to the smooth running and success of the conference. Plenary speakers and other participants were generously supported by the National Health Service Women's Unit, the Wellcome Trust and the British Academy. We are grateful to those bodies for their help in promoting nursing history. Robert Dingwall, Helen Meller and Julian Robinson were unstinting in their contributions to the early organization of the conference and in chairing sessions. The staff of the Department of Nursing and Midwifery Studies gave generously of their time and expertise in chairing sessions. We are grateful to Veronica James, Mary Chapple, John Fletcher, Mark Avis, Sara Owen, Chris Glazebrook, Tony Thompson, Linda East, Liz Hart. Hilary Marland, Paul Weindling, Shula Marks, Olive Stephenson, Peggy Nuttall chaired plenary papers and for that we wish to thank them. We benefited from the superb stewarding skills of the students from the Department of Nursing and Midwifery Studies. We wish to thank all the 235 participants who presented papers and attended the conference for their enthusiasm which contributed in no small way to a scholarly and supportive atmosphere.

Grateful thanks are due to Sage Publications and the *Western Journal of Nursing Research* for allowing us to republish Barbara Brush's article, 'The Rockefeller agenda for American/Philippines nursing relations' (Chapter 3) and to Blackwell Science Inc. for permission to publish extracts from Geertje Boschma, 'The meaning of holism in nursing: historical shifts in holistic nursing ideas', *Public Health Nursing*, 1994, 11, 5, pp. 324–30.

Introduction

INFUSING INFLUENCE

A quiet revolution has been sweeping through the writing of nursing history over the past decade. Two new journals, *The International History of Nursing Journal* and *Nursing History Review* attest to this trend. Nursing history is slowly being transformed from an internalist and triumphalist form of professional apologetics to a robust and reflective area of scholarship. It is attracting attention and research interest from a broad spectrum of scholars drawn from women's history, labour history, history of medicine, sociology and, of course, nursing itself. The collection presented here reveals the increasingly gender and politically aware perspectives that are emerging from the cross-fertilization of ideas and interdisciplinary and international contact between social historians of medicine, nursing, historians of gender and the politics of welfare. It demonstrates the important contribution that historians of nursing can make to setting a new intellectual and political agenda for nurses, one in which the politics of nursing and welfare can fuse and flourish.

The multidisciplinary and international range of perspectives included in this volume reflects the growing richness of nursing history's intellectual identity. History provides an important filter through which insights and analyses drawn from other disciplines can reach nursing audiences. This, in turn, will help to expand interest in nursing's history on the part of new constituencies, shifting the shape and form of the field in the process. Christopher Maggs, in discussing contemporary practice and concerns in nursing history, raised the question: 'Is there something that can be called nursing history'?[1] The answer to that question is probably that it depends. What 'counts' as nursing history is contingent upon the dynamics that define the relations between authors and audiences who form the intellectual community of nursing history, and indeed of any field of enquiry, at any given time. As with the history of medicine, nursing has a hybrid historiographical heritage, one that is porous and permeable to a matrix of influences.

TRENDS AND THEMES

The present volume attempts to build on the historiographical challenge set by Celia Davies's mould-breaking edited collection and Christopher Maggs' sequel of more than a decade ago.[2] It shares some of the features and aspirations discussed by Kathryn McPherson and Meryn Stuart in their review essay of the 'new' historiography of Canadian nursing.[3] While some chapters treat traditional topics in fresh ways, other themes, notably those of race, class, gender, internationalism and imperialism especially, are brought into sharper focus. While some of the chapters are the products of mature research, others derive from those who have more recently embarked upon their research careers and whom we were keen to encourage. As well as including a range of expertise, we have selected contributions which reflect the international nature of historical research in nursing. Thus case studies from India, South Africa, Australia, the USA, Philippines, Germany, Scotland, as well as England, are included. The chapters included here highlight the role that politics plays in understanding the history of nursing and the reciprocal role that history has to play in the political education of nurses. This, of course, is hardly a new role for nursing history to play. Political interests have exerted an enduring influence upon the writing of nursing history. Many of the early nursing histories were written by nurse leaders and their sympathizers operating as extensions of their campaigns for nurses' registration and suffrage.[4] Accounts of nursing history are revealing of how nursing work is perceived and defined at any given point in time. Take the early nurse historians, Lavinia Dock and Adelaide Nutting, for example. Their association of nursing with the instinctual basis of caring celebrated in Peter Kropotkin's *Mutual Aid* drew an analogy between the biological and social worlds.[5] Nutting and Dock were keen to associate nursing with the evolutionary characteristics of altruism and co-operation, attributed by Kropotkin to the survival of superior species. Thus history was used to justify the 'scientific' basis of nursing values. But history has also been used by nurse historians to legitimize claims to professionalism, the independent development of nursing from medicine and the pursuit of autonomy by nurses.[6] Only with the rise of a more critical rather than congratulatory approach to nursing's claims to professionalism was this assumption questioned. Revisionist accounts that examined nursing's failure to obtain occupational closure and exposed the heterogeneous social origins of nurse recruitment revealed the problematic nature of claims to professionalism.[7] Most recently accounts have been refined into more gender aware perspectives.[8] These have analysed nursing's claims to professionalism as paradigmatic of the contradictions inherent within the gendered nature of professions.[9]

Recurrent crises in nurse recruitment and historical analyses of the social composition of the nursing workforce have raised crucial questions about the therapeutic effectiveness of nursing care. Underlying such concerns are the problematics that attach to the nurse's role as a social catalyst in care, a cross-class and cultural conduit into the lives and social spaces of groups otherwise beyond the reach of agents of social authority. A key theme informing the present volume is the extent to which nurses represent extensions of, or challenges to, the authority with which they are invested. Notwithstanding appropriation of a rhetoric of advocacy, whose interests is it possible for nurses to represent? This raises the vexed question of social symmetry and the extent to which nurses can claim expertise in caring for patients whose social origins are distinct from their own. Does the cultural specificity of nursing undermine attempts to theorize nursing and health care in universalist terms, terms in which the nature of care itself is contested?

CONTENT AND CONTEXT

The chapters presented here draw upon a rich vein of source material both oral and documentary, traversing wide and deep tranches of time and space. Government papers, private foundation records, literary sources, and those emanating from professional associations are all included to illuminate the light and dark sides of nursing's history. What each of the contributions reinforces is that nursing cannot be understood in its own terms but against the background of the social, political, economic and cultural context in which it subsists. Characteristic of this 'new' historiography of nursing is its exposure of the segmented and stratified nature of the nursing workforce; one which is divided across race, class and gender lines, reflecting the economic and political hierarchies of society more generally. That nursing is shaped by the context in which it subsists is illustrated by each chapter in turn but perhaps most poignantly by Hilde Steppe's essay on nursing in the Third Reich. Hilde Steppe vividly reconstructs the compliance of nurses with the ethos and practice of Nazi medicine. She dissects out the rationalizations Nazi nurses used to justify their deadly actions as a case study of nursing within a totalitarian political regime. In particular Hilde Steppe draws attention to the double-bind in which nurses are placed when finally nursing is valued within a political culture but, as it transpires, for all too sinister reasons. The role of nurses, usually portrayed as one of the guardian angels of human rights, is contradicted so deeply by this episode in history, it raises profound questions about the capacity of nurses to act as patients' advocates, their 'resistance' role within change, one that is so vaunted in contemporary nursing theory and policy.

Shula Marks continues this theme of nursing history as the history of the present in her chapter on the nursing profession in South Africa and the making of apartheid. In her essay Shula Marks argues that the history of the nursing profession provides a powerful metaphor for the study of South African society. Underlying such a history lie deep and riveting tensions generated by the universalist ethos of nursing and racial, class and gender-based fears surrounding images of white (female) nurses' hands on black (male) patients' bodies. Marks' chapter considers the implications of the racially segmented professionalizing politics of South African nursing for the 'new' South Africa and the identity politics within which nursing, as one of the most important occupations for women in South Africa, is enmeshed.

Barbara Brush elaborates this theme of yesterday's history as today's policy in her essay on the long-term sequelae of the Rockefeller Foundation's exploits in the Philippines during the 1920s. She argues that the Rockefeller agenda for nursing in the Philippines has repercussions for the racialized recruitment of nurses into areas of shortage in the USA today. Rather than providing culturally sensitive health care and nurse education in the Philippines in the 1920s the Rockefeller Foundation set in train a series of cultural changes which unwittingly created a pipeline of labour from the Philippines to short-staffed American hospitals. The long-term legacy of the Rockefeller's imperialist initiatives are examined as a case study in the colonialist politics of the caste-system in nursing.

The interface between imperial and indigenous medical and nursing practice is explored by Rosemary Fitzgerald in her examination of British Protestant women medical missionaries between 1870 and 1970. At the heart of the Indian missionary enterprise lay the desire to bring Western forms of medical aid and nurse training to the women of India. The consequences of this 'movement' are discussed in terms of their implications for the professionalization of nursing in India, the complex relations between gender, empire, women's diverse experience of colonialism and the British bequest of medical mission work for women in post-colonial India.

Counteracting the dominance of nurse historians' fascination with general nursing, Harriet Deacon moves into the margins of care in her examination of mental, chronic-sick pauper and leper nursing in the Robben Island General Infirmary between 1846 and 1931. Contrary to the conventional imagery of nurses as single, twenty-something, female and educated, staff at Robben Island were mostly married, inexperienced and middle-aged, in the 1850s. Moreover patients continued to assist in nursing lepers and the chronic sick until 1892, when the latter were removed. Patients as well as nurses broke the mould. Far from being the supine supplicating souls of contemporary nursing discourse, Robben Island patients were recalcitrant and intractable. So much so that they proved too much for the Nightingale-trained contingent of nurses from Kimberley to tolerate and manage. The inducements of mental nurse training were insufficient to raise the retention rates for staff and the increasing influx of black and prison patients after the 1890s reinforced the rough-and-ready image of the Island and the nursing work within it as mainly a male preserve.

The importance of men in nursing is discussed in Angela Cushing's essay on the dynamics of caring in Australia prior to the introduction of female nursing in 1868. The first settler nurses in Australia were men brought over on the ships of the British

Admiralty and the contractors who assisted in the convict transportation process. The tensions between the caring work of men
with and as convicts and the 'reformed' military model of female
nursing imported by Lucy Osburn from Miss Nightingale are
discussed. The tensions in gender and class relations in colonial
Australian nursing are considered against the background of the
shifting dynamic between the imperial impulse and indigenous
identity in Australian nursing.

The contested nature and construction of nursing work is discussed by Barbara Mortimer in her analysis of pre-reform nursing
in Edinburgh. Using Census and Post Office records, she tracks
the organization of nurses and nursing work in the mid-nineteenth
century. She teases out the social and economic dynamics driving
nursing work in institutions and 'private' practice. Although some
nurses worked co-operatively, many worked independently,
especially those who headed up households. Mortimer's paper
casts a rare beam of light into the organization and survival
strategies of nurses in Edinburgh, whose famous medical school
has eclipsed historical analysis of nursing. Her paper begins to
redress the historiographical bias in favour of medical practice
in Edinburgh, bringing Scotland within the sights of the nurse
historian's 'gaze'.

Language provides a powerful vehicle for socialization. In his
chapter on professionalization, gender and the language of training, Tom Olson analyses the tension between nursing textbooks
and records of training in communicating occupational culture in
nursing. Contrary to the high-minded ideals of contemporary
claimants to a tradition of caring as the defining essence of nursing, Olson exposes the contradictory evidence from the values
enshrined in the training records of a mid-West American training
school between 1915 and 1937. Rather than confirming the ideological and practical purity of 'caring' within nurse training, the
reward system reinforced values of handling, managing and controlling individuals and situations with the intention of producing
neat, finished appearing work.

The role of ideology lies at the heart of Geertje Boschma's
paper on holism, which nursing championed as an alternative to
the biomedical model of care and hence medical subordination
from the late nineteenth century until the present. American
nursing perceived itself as adding a psycho-social dimension to
the medical model, an area of expertise which was 'gendered' and

provided the means by which nurses could assert an independent identity from medicine. Boschma argues however that the championing of holism by nurses had a paradoxical twist; defining nursing oppositionally to medicine did not remove the dependence of nursing upon medicine for its identity.

The politics of paradox are continued in Judith Godden's paper on nursing as philanthropic work in Australia between 1880 and 1930. Godden argues that when feminists and others have championed the cause of nurses in demanding improved working conditions, rank and file nurses and their leaders have often rejected such offers of help. What nursing sympathizers deemed exploitation, nurse leaders have, at times, viewed as professionalism, dedication and duty. Godden maintains that early nurse leaders walked a political tightrope between creating a gendered space in which women's expertise could flourish while setting standards of professionalism which would qualify nurses for the rewards that accrued to professional work. She concludes that political and material costs of the leadership legacy of those early nurse strategists are still being paid today.

Recruitment crises and episodes of acute shortage of nursing labour are notorious catalysts for reform programmes in nursing. Glenda Strachan's essay on nurse recruitment during World War II in Australia explores the paradox of nursing's exclusion from government regulations to attract more women into the workforce by improving conditions, in spite of dire shortages. Contrary to the policy adopted for doctors and female workers, nurses were directed into nursing and domestic service. Some nurses retaliated by striking in protest at what they perceived as authoritarian action on the part of the government. Strachan explores and attempts to explain the government action in the context of the wartime regulation of medical and female labour.

The contested nature of nursing as a career is discussed by Sarah Abrams and Jenny Maxwell in their essays on the Rockefeller Foundation activities and nursing in the 1920s and child welfare policy in the late nineteenth–early twentieth centuries respectively. Taking primarily a sociological tack, Abrams considers the role of the Rockefeller Foundation in underwriting competing claims to professional jurisdiction by different professional groups such as social workers and public health nurses during the 1920s. Further forms of accommodation were required by nurses to find a niche within the scientific framework of

Rockefeller philanthropy. Their task was double-edged, being concerned with articulating an altruistic version of women's mission while at the same time using the language of science to legitimize nurses' claims to jurisdiction in public health work.

Continuing this theme of regulation, Jenny Maxwell argues that the conventional dichotomy between socio-legal and medico-social approaches to child care policy is an artificial one. Whereas the socio-legal perspective focuses upon the coercive power of the state to intervene in the regulation of private life and protect care for children as either victims or potential victims of family abuse, breakdown or neglect, the medico-social perspective emphasizes the role of state intervention in providing for the physical, educational and health needs of children and families. Rather than perceiving these two approaches as separate or distinctive, Jenny Maxwell argues that child care and welfare should be conceived as elements of the wider goals of social regulation.

In her essay on the politics of career development for women, Ellen Baer compares the problems and potential of the 'equal' rights or 'difference' approaches to career development for nurses. Baer delineates the major dilemma for the most recent feminist movement in the USA, which has been whether to advocate for women's position as equal to or different from men's. She contends that feminists who promote the entry of women into careers formerly dominated by men implicitly demean traditional feminine roles. As a nurse, Baer argues that her inclination as well as her political preference is to empower traditional female roles such as nursing rather than witness the diversion of talented women away from nursing. A number of strategies are proposed to counteract the trend which appears to favour male-dominated professions.

Finally, mirroring the concluding chapter by Julia Foster and Julia Shepherd in Celia Davies's ground-breaking edited collection of more than a decade ago, Lesley Hall takes a more recent look at nursing's archives through an excursion in the archival deposits on nursing held at the Wellcome Institute and elsewhere. She considers the historical record created by the different strands of the nursing profession and the use to which that record has and can be put.

NOTES

1 C. Maggs, 'Nursing history: contemporary practice and contemporary concerns', in C. Maggs (ed.), *Nursing History: The State of the Art*, London, Croom Helm, 1987, p. 2.

2 C. Davies (ed.), *Rewriting Nursing History*, London, Croom Helm, 1980; C. Maggs, op. cit.

3 See K. McPherson and M. Stuart, 'Writing nursing history in Canada: issues and approaches', *Canadian Bulletin of Medical History*, 1994, vol. 11, pp. 3–22.

4 For further discussion on these points see A.M. Rafferty, 'Historical perspectives', in B. Vaughan and K. Robinson (eds), *Knowledge for Nursing Practice*, Oxford, Butterworth Heinemann, 1992, pp. 26–41.

5 P. Kropotkin, *Mutual Aid: A Factor in Human Evolution*, London, Heinemann, 1902.

6 See Rafferty, op. cit., pp. 34–6.

7 See the collection of conference papers in D. Stapleton and C. Welch (eds), *Critical Issues in American Nursing in the Twentieth Century: Perspectives and Case Studies*, New York, Foundation of the New York State Nurses Association, 1994.

8 B. Abel-Smith, *A History of the Nursing Profession*, London, Heinemann, 1960; C. Davies, op. cit.; C. Maggs, *The Origins of General Nursing*, London, Croom Helm, 1983; C. Maggs, 1987, op. cit.

9 See A. Witz, *Professions and Patriarchy*, London, Routledge, 1992; C. Davies, *Gender and the Professional Predicament of Nursing*, Milton Keynes, Open University Press, 1995.

Chapter 1

Nursing under totalitarian regimes: the case of National Socialism

Hilde Steppe

This chapter presents a small extract taken from my efforts over the last fifteen years to deal with a portion of our nursing history – the period of German National Socialism.

When I began my research, I was interested in filling in a gap in our history. It quickly became clear that this was not a normal gap but a deep-seated taboo; touching it produced not so much a sense of satisfaction but instead mistrust, rejection and fear. This research has meant not only dealing with the history of my profession, but also dealing with the history of my parents' and teachers' generation and the history of my country where I was born in a refugee camp and later grew up. This research raised questions about my personal relationship to this period of history and my own defence mechanisms against the reality of nursing under National Socialism.

Opening myself to this process of reflection means that this work is not finished for me and so I can only share with you the present state of that knowledge.

In order to reconstruct this period of time I have analysed primary data found in a number of public and private archives. I have also used the methods of oral history by analysing the accounts given in nearly 200 written or personal interviews.

In this chapter I will address four questions:

1 What was the special function of nursing during National Socialism?
2 How were nursing tasks performed by nurses at that time?
3 How, after 1945, did nursing deal with this period of history?
4 What lessons can we draw from this period of history?

In order to answer the question of the specific function of nursing, it is necessary to briefly describe the organization of German nursing before 1933.

During the second half of the nineteenth century, nursing was declared to be the ideal occupation for middle-class women and was completely reorganized. Up until that time, two relatively independent care systems had exisited – one, that of religious orders which based their care on the Christian concept of love for one's neighbour, and the other of care for the sick by paid orderlies. The system of paid orderlies (*Lohnwartsystem*) evolved mainly in the Protestant areas of Germany after the Reformation, since the Catholic orders had been disbanded during the course of the Reformation. It was not until the first half of the nineteenth century that Catholic orders began to be refounded. At the same time, Lutheran nursing (*Diakonissenrankenpflege*) was developing on the Protestant side.[1,2,3] The socio-economic upheavals of the nineteenth century broke up these two systems, and a third branch of nursing emerged, that of independent nurses. The collapse of these two systems can be attributed to a number of factors. First, industrialization dissolved the system of domestic and family care and necessitated forms of public provision, like hospitals, in ever-increasing numbers. Second, the rapid development of medicine, which had become increasingly oriented towards the natural sciences, required at least passably well-trained and willing assistant staff to undertake all the activities in the field of diagnosis and therapy that had now become 'unscientific'. Third, the development of civil welfare had supplemented and increasingly replaced the ecclesiastical caritas. Fourth, there was a struggle for emancipation, mainly among middle-class women, which had to be directed into socially acceptable channels by men. Fourth, as a result of the wars which took place in the nineteenth century, and under the influence, primarily, of the work of Florence Nightingale, it was declared that optimal medical care for the wounded should be a national duty of prime importance. Lastly, the final overcoming of feudalism in Europe paved the way for the establishment of bourgeoise society with its fixed moral and gender-specifice codes.[4]

By the nineneenth century the task in hand was to react to the increased demand for nursing, which, in concrete terms, meant going beyond the ecclesiastical organizations and establishing the occupation as 'socially acceptable'. However, this could only be accomplished by a successful appeal to a particular social class whose members would feel a strong commitment to the values represented by nursing. In the nineteenth century it was bourgeois women, in the main, who presented themselves as suitable for the task, since they had internalized the values of female morality. The demands of the bourgeois women's movement to realize a gender-specific division of labour in the public sector meant opening up occupations to them which corresponded with the 'female nature'. These demands were ideally suited to the establishment of the nursing occupation, since this occupation was guaranteed to fit well into the fixed frame of the patriarchal world picture. Independent nursing gradually established itself, actively promoted as it was by middle-class women who saw it as a way of entering the world outside the home and therefore as a step towards emancipation. It was also supported by male medical doctors who saw nursing as the position in health care allocated to women. The price that women had to pay for the support of men was the subordination of nursing to the absolute domination of medicine and the accompanying surrender of any shred of independence. Serving, giving of oneself, self-sacrifice and obedience became the intrinsic values of middle-class women's nursing and so constituted the perfect professional ethical pitfall for all nurses. Self-awareness and self-determination were declared to be inappropriate and irreconcilable with the 'ideal' professional posture and stance.

In looking at this complex process of professional development, there are five main characteristics which can be identified:

1 The absolute subordination of nursing to medicine, where the one exists only by virtue of its relationship with the other;
2 The gender-specific nature of the nursing ideal; the complete intermingling of personal and professional qualifications resulting in an inability to develop any professional distance;
3 The limitless and never-ending boundaries of professional reponsibility;
4 The splintering of nursing into competing ideological groups;
5 The hostile stance of many nurses towards a collective occupational identity. As middle-class women, nurses did not want to be associated with the demands of the labour movement since such demands conflicted with nurses' own view of themselves as individual professionals.

The effects of these vocation-specific traits culminated in a lack of professional independence, disagreement about professional policy, uncertainty about the scope and content of nursing, low societal recognition reflected in a lack of occupational security, and an unattainable constellation of professional ideals which, above all, resulted in a radical denial of their own needs.

Only against this backdrop is it possible to understand the developments in nursing which began in 1933 and the reaction of the nurses themselves to these developments.

I return now to the first question I posed, that of the specific function of nursing in National Socialism, which I want to clarify with respect to the following aspects: the incorporation of nursing into the National Socialist policies for health and for women; the terms of reference with regard to professional nursing practice; the tasks allocated to nursing; and the significance of nursing for the state.

National Socialist health policy was marked by extreme polarities, that is, simultaneous selection (of the best) and extermination (of the undesirable). Ideologically, policy was based on the concept of social hygiene and racial purity (eugenics). This political platform was not unique to the Nazis, but could be found, not only in Germany but also in other countries, as early as the late nineteenth century and was expressed in the ideology of social Darwinism.[5] From this theory the Nazis took several central elements: the biologistic view of state and society, the idea of total state control, the necessity for propagation or active promotion of racially valuable characteristics and the elimination of the racially inferior classes, and the notion of the survival of the fittest.[6]

This led to a far-reaching paradigm shift in health care and to specific political action beginning in 1933. For example, in 1934 the law for the prevention of hereditary diseases was passed. This law set out the framework for compulsory sterilization. The humanistic and Christian healing tradition in which the focus was on the individual was sacrificed to the overarching needs of the health of the whole nation. The individual was now valued only for his contribution to the whole.[7] Nazis reasoned that if an individual could not contribute to the whole, then this individual had no right to care by society; on the contrary, society had the right and the duty to banish this socially unfit person in order to preserve the health of all. The slogan for public health was 'Vorsorge statt Fürsorge' which translates roughly as 'prevention not protection', 'cure not care' or 'public health not sentimental humanitarianism'.[8]

These health policies were binding for all health professionals. Nurses, who were numerically the strongest group in health care, were given special attention from the beginning. They were to play an important role in the health education of the people through their continual contact with the sick. They were also involved in both of the National Socialist extremes – in supporting the 'worthy' and in destroying the lives of those deemed 'unworthy'.

The Head Office for Public Welfare issued the following declaration in 1936:

> In the future nursing should be not only concerned with the sick and suffering, it should consist not ONLY in caring for the ill, in relieving the effects of poverty or current need. It must go further. Nursing must lead the people in questions of health. It is a nurse who should carry out the will of the State in the health education of the people.[9]

In addition to this not unimportant role in health policy, the professional structure of nursing fitted in very well with the gendered National Socialist image of the 'natural task of the woman in the state'. From our perspective today, the Nazi women's policy seems a very complex and contradictory construction; it has not yet been adequately researched. However, we can say there was no uniform policy that applied to all women since it was their racial identity which was the most important factor. Every regulation designed to benefit women automatically excluded a number of women who were seen to be racially unworthy.[10]

For the Nazi state, the ideal woman was the mother, the 'bearer of blood and race', so that her biological ability to give birth was also evaluated on the basis of her racial purity.[11] Also the working woman was seen positively, as long as she was in a job which was appropriate for her as a woman and which was seen as serving the people. Bertha Braun of the National Socialism women's movement summed up the mood of 'maternalism'. She argued that:

> such phrases as 'spiritual motherhood' and 'expanded motherliness' could only mean a transference of the idea of selflessness and self-sacrifice in all areas of life, not only in natural

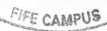

motherhood. The authority of motherhood was based simply on the awe that every selfless sacrifice calls forth.[12]

Gertrud Scholtz-Kling, the Third Reich's Women's Leader, stated the basis for women's work on 26 October 1934 at a political rally:

> Women will find their place at all times and in all places where the work they are given is in the right relationship to their strength. Whether that strength is on an intellectual level or on another level is completely irrelevant. In every case, work achievement must always correspond to the strength and the inner spiritual orientation of the woman, and then all conflicts cease to exist.[13]

Thus, true motherhood was possible at home and at work and women's vocations met the ideal insofar as they incorporated motherly aspects. The motherly vocation of nursing fitted this image quite well and therefore received public recognition. An advertising brochure from 1938 stated that 'next to the task of motherhood a woman has no more beautiful and feminine an occupation than in the profession of a nurse'.[14]

The dual importance of nursing both as an ideal profession for women and as an influential factor in national health policy can also be seen in the state's efforts to define the boundaries of nursing work and tasks. The stated intention of these measures was, on the one hand, to promote uniformity and tighten up organizational structures, and on the other, to conform with the professional concepts and content of the newly emerging nursing organizations. Toward this end the *NS-Schwesternshaft*, Nazi Nursing Organization, which was to serve as a model for all other nursing organizations, was founded in 1934 as a sub-organization of the Nazi party. As Erna Mach, a nurse and leader of the Nazi Nursing Organization, declared:

> The primary task of training nurses in accordance with the wishes of Adolf Hitler and of joining together into a National Socialist organisation is uniquely the task of the NS Nursing Association. All other nursing in the future will have to orient itself to the thought and methods of this Association.[15]

All the larger organizations involved in nursing (the German Red Cross, Catholic and Protestant organizations, and independent organizations) were summarily subsumed into a *Reichsfachschaft* which operated under the auspices of the Ministry of the Interior which was a more or less state-controlled umbrella organization. Men and women were segregated into separate organizations. Unions, socialist and communist nursing organizations were forcibly disbanded and their members required to join one of the recognized organizations. Jewish nurses were not admitted into either the umbrella organization or the Nazi Nursing Association, but neither was their organization disbanded. It was retained in order to continue to provide nursing care for Jewish people.

The many hitherto independent groups were amalgamated in 1936 into the *Reichsbund Deutscher Schwestern und Pflegerinnen*, the *Reichsbund* of German Nurses. Their members wore a blue uniform in contrast with the brown uniforms of the Nazi nurses. In 1942 the blue nurses and the brown nurses were joined into the 'National Socialist Reichsbund of German Nurses'. Responsibility for nursing was delegated to the *Nationale Sozialist Volkswohlfahrt* (NSV), the National Socialist Welfare Organization, the largest organization in the Nazi Party. With regard to questions related to nurses' training, nurses came under the jurisdiction of the *Hauptampt für Volksgesundheit*, Head Office of Public Health of the Nazi Party, all of whose key positions were occupied by doctors.

The attempts of a few nursing organizations to maintain their independence failed because the allocation of jobs and job promotion were tied to membership of one of the recognized organizations. In order to further control access to, and provision of, public services a *Warnkartei* ('warning card file') was created which soon came to be used extensively as a selection instrument to exclude from public service all persons deemed 'unfit'. Those who had been excluded from public service were eligible only to work in private institutions, usually church-related.

In order to deal with the chronic shortage of nursing personnel, huge advertising campaigns were conducted in which the social importance of nursing was stressed. An advertising brochure of the time stated that 'Men serve with weapons ... women serve by watching over and caring for life at its basis, in a motherly, sisterly way, using all the tenderness and strength which nature has given them in order to fulfil this task'.[16]

A central component of the creation of a uniform nursing profession was the passage of the first National Nursing Act in

1938. Herein the tasks of nursing were defined for the first time. Training was standardized at one and a half years, and a practical year thereafter was required for licensing. This Act marked the formal integration of nursing into the Nazi system. Thereafter only Aryan women could become German nurses. But Jewish nurses could still be trained; they received a card stating their identity. The Act did not apply to psychiatry so in this branch no uniform training course or examination existed.

One of the most important changes in nursing was the expansion of duties which evolved out of the Nazi health policies. For the first time since the reorganization of nursing in the nineteenth century, nursing was allocated its own field of work, that of public health (*Volksgesundheitspflege*).

The new-found status of nursing was described in bold and militaristic terms by one contemporary:

> Just as, for example, German doctors were given entirely new, expanded responsibilities through National Socialism, so, for us Socialists, it cannot be enough for the task of a nurse to define herself only as the assistant of the doctor in treating and caring for the sick and, in addition, to the best of her ability, to care for the physical and emotional well-being of those entrusted to her and to take part in a more or less harmonious nursing association. For us a nurse is also to be a political soldier.[17]

In public health, nurses took over responsibilities for counselling, supervision and instruction in health maintenance for the population. The nurse gave advice on stocking up on reserves of food and household supplies, made recommendations on cooking recipes, encouraged thrift, and made decisions on further health measures such as sending children out to the country or reporting 'deviant' behaviour. Because of the importance of these functions, they were to be carried out as far as possible only by Nazi nurses. The existing community nursing service which was under the control of the churches was gradually replaced by Nazi district nursing offices. Caring for the sick in hospitals remained one of the chief responsibilities of nurses. Here, nurses from all associations were employed including a small number of male nurses.

The nursing care of the Nazi party and all its sub-groups was exclusively the responsibility of Nazi nurses. The politicians were also interested in having sufficient numbers of nurses available in case of war. When other countries were occupied and conquered, nurses were sent there to provide nursing care and public education. Taking part in crimes against humanity was also a task of nurses in National Socialism.

In summary, it can be said that nursing was an important factor in public health policy, expressed in the tasks allocated to it. Nurses were involved in nursing activities at all levels of health care and in the related Nazi party organizations. The status of the nursing profession was enhanced. For the first time uniform standards were developed which gave the members of the profession some sense of security. For these reasons it is possible to understand why most of those I interviewed reported that 1933 was a positive turning point in their career, a time of 'discipline' and the expansion of possibilities for advancement in their profession. The ambiguity of this enhanced status becomes apparent only on closer examination of the responsibilities of the nursing profession. In fact, nurses were fully under the control of the Nazi party system of health care and Nazi party discipline. As before, medical doctors determined the nature of the nursing profession; in addition, the professional ethic was still based on obedience, sacrifice and selfless service. Therefore there was a smooth transition from the old to the new ideology. The devaluation of the nurse as an independent person continued in that only her anonymous and self-sacrificial service to her people was honoured. Nurses were still not seen as individual persons with their own wishes and needs; on the contrary, their sacrifice of their own personality was declared to be their contribution and was rewarded only trivially. This ambiguous message, namely that only through self-denial could nurses participate in great accomplishments, appears to have been successful, for without the contribution of over 100,000 nurses National Socialist health policy could never have been carried out.

Turning next to the second question posed at the start of this chapter I want to look at the issue of how nurses perceived and carried out their tasks during the Nazi era. In more concrete terms, I wish to address the question of which categories of nurse can be discerned. For the purpose of analysis I have identified five groups – the enthusiasts, the conformists, the obedient, the persecuted and the resisters.

For the 'enthusiasts', the year 1933 marked a new era which they greatly welcomed. Some of them had already been committed National Socialists since the 1920s and had organized themselves into National Socialist self-help groups that rendered first aid to the paramilitary storm troopers (*Sturmabteilung* – SA), following street fights.[18] They were said to be the germ core of the later NS nursing organization, although several veterans were not promoted to higher positions after 1933 because they were too openly far right-wing extremists. After her training, the NS-nurse publicly took an oath that declared her bonds with the National Socialist ideology:

> I solemnly swear that I will be steadfastly faithful and obedient to Adolf Hitler, my Führer (my leader). I promise to fulfil my duties, wherever I may be designated to work, faithfully and conscientiously as a national-socialist nurse in service to the national community, so help me God.[19]

On the assumption that all members of the NS-nursing organization can be reckoned among the enthusiasts, they represent just under 10 per cent of all nurses up to 1939.[20]

The 'conformists' are defined as those who, prior to 1933, had not expressed their approval of National Socialism and who afterwards, for various reasons, at least outwardly came to terms with it. The conformists represent the largest group of nurses and, according to official pronouncements, all those organizations which had not been immediately dissolved by force must be counted in this group (but not, of course, all of their members!). The Protestant nursing orders had already united in a *Diakoniegemeinschaft*, a diaconate association, in 1933 and had sent Hitler a telegram on the occasion of their public rally in November 1933:

> Being overwhelmed by the saving grace of God given to our dearly beloved nation once again through your hand, and conscious of their mutual responsibility for the motherly duties which millions are waiting for, the diaconate associations united within the Reich's professional association of German nurses now meeting at the teachers' association's house pledge their willing sacrificial service and eternal fidelity to our God-given Fuehrer![21]

The nurses belonging to the nursing organization of the German Red Cross took the following oath:

I swear to be faithful to the Führer of the German Reich, Adolf Hitler. I vow obedience and performance of my duties regarding the task of the German Red Cross on the orders of my superiors. So help me God.[22]

On 15 May 1933, the following text was printed on the cover of the magazine *Unterm Lazaruskrenz* (*Under Lazarus' Cross*), the information bulletin of the *Berufsorganisation der Krankenpflegerinnen Deutschland*, the professional organization of German nurses (the trade association founded by Agnes Karll):

It is obvious that the association whose members are German nurses is solidly behind the new government. We want to take part in the great tasks lying before us and those which will arise out of this new era.[23]

The 'Catholic Nurses' Association of Germany' (*Catholischer Schwesternerband Deutschlands*) took part in the professional association of the German Reich right from the beginning. However, they complained about the lack of co-operation of other Catholic unions. It was only from 1937 that the Caritas organization was represented at meetings of nurses' associations by a nun and a lay Catholic nurse.[24]

This large group of conformists can best be characterized by the following statements made in the interviews: 'I tried to continue to do my best.' 'I thought I could prevent something worse, if I participated.' 'Of course, I considered many things not to be right, however, what should I have done?' 'I merely went on fulfilling my duties.' Many of those whom I interviewed described changes in the practice of their profession, for example, dismissal of Jewish colleagues and spying by party members; they spoke too about their fears and their rejection of the new government. However, they thought they were too weak to change anything and therefore tried simply to carry on doing their work.

The 'obedient' also carried on doing their work and followed the orders given to them. All those who took part in the crimes against humanity out of obedience can be counted in this group. Even today, we know only very little about the specific nursing aspects in the destruction of lives deemed to be 'unworthy of living'. It is certain, however, that female and male nurses were involved in all stages of extermination. They worked in psychiatric institutions from which patients were sent to their death, they worked in the murder institutions where thousands were gassed; some were even sent to work in several institutions, one after the other. Nurses killed patients in the mental institutions during the phase described as rampant euthanasia (1941–45). The selection of victims was no longer centrally organized but was carried out in each institution directly. And in obediently carrying out this murderous task they tried to remain good nurses. This perversion of caring concern at the moment of death became clear for me in the statement made by nurse Anna G.:

> Patients who were strong enough sat themselves up in bed; we laid an extra pillow under the heads of the others in order to lift them up a little. In giving them the dissolved substance, I proceeded with great compassion. I had told the patients earlier that they had to have a little treatment. Obviously, I could only tell this little tale to those patients who were conscious enough to understand. In giving them the drink, I took them in my arms and caressed them. If they did not empty the glass, for example, because it tasted so bitter, then I encouraged them by saying they had drunk so much of it, they should drink the rest of it, because otherwise the treatment would not be complete. Some of them were so persuaded by my encouragement that they finished the glass completely. With others, we fed them by spoonfuls. As I said before, the way we proceeded was determined by the patient's behaviour and condition.[25]

This same nurse later answered a question in the course of her interrogation by saying:

> I would not have robbed a bank or committed a theft, because that simply is not done. Apart from that, a theft would not have been part of my job.[26]

In the course of the later proceedings, most nurses justified the murder as obedience to the doctors.

> From the beginning, that is, from the time when I was a nursing student, I learned to show unquestioning obedience towards the superior and older nurses. I assume the fact of absolute obedience within nursing circles is generally known, so that I do not need to go into details here.[27]

It was and it is my conviction that it is one of the most important duties of any nurse to follow absolutely the doctor's orders.[28]

The obedient therefore did what they were told to do, and they did it even if they personally did not approve of the act. In the words of one nurse:

Personally, however, I was not of the opinion that such human beings should be killed; I had previously looked after these seriously ill persons with loving care for many years. Personally, I was of the opinion that, if it were ordered by the doctor and if it had been ordered by the government . . . then it must be right.[29]

This part of nursing's execution of tasks certainly can be seen as one of the darkest chapters in the history of nursing. Even if the number of those who were obedient in this way was small – the precise figure is still unknown – it does represent a crucial factor in the practical application of National Socialist health policy.

Unfortunately, since their history has not yet been written, the least is known to date about the group of nurses who were 'persecuted'. Belonging to this group were all those female and male colleagues who were not allowed to go on doing their work for political, religious, sexist or racist reasons, those who were spied upon, betrayed and persecuted, those who were dismissed, arrested, interned and murdered, and those who had to emigrate and were given refuge in other nations. Today, there are nurses who had to flee from Germany or Austria who live in Great Britain, where they have actively taken part in the development of the nursing profession. Many nurses of Jewish origin were removed to concentration camps, where they tried to keep up nursing care, as has been recorded, for example, by Resi Weglein for Theresienstadt. Weglein lists the names of thirteen Austrian, fourteen German and two Czech nurses, of whom only seven survived. The others were killed in Auschwitz.[30]

The history of Jewish nursing in Germany, too, which represented an important part of health care and nursing, has not yet been adequately researched. However, there was also a group of 'resisters' – female and male nurses who did not conform but resisted National Socialism for political, humanistic or religious reasons. There is little trace of their activities. To date only about fifty female and male nurses have been recorded by name, although their total number was almost certainly higher. The following two must stand on behalf of all of them.

Sister M. Restituta (Helene Kafka) was an Austrian nun who worked as a theatre sister near Vienna. She was an unyielding fighter against National Socialism and did not let anything overturn her firm beliefs. For example, acting in contempt of an express prohibition, she hung the Holy Cross in sick-rooms and distributed a patriotic soldier's poem which suggested desertion. In 1942 she was arrested in the operating theatre; there was hardly anyone who spoke up on her behalf after she was sentenced to death. She was executed, in March 1943, at 49 years of age.

Emmy Dörfel, a Communist, was arrested for the first time in 1933. She emigrated to France and worked in the medical service with the International Brigades in Spain, was interned in France afterwards and later returned to Germany. She was arrested and taken away to the concentration camp Ravensbrück. In 1945 she managed to escape. Today she lives in eastern Berlin.

When we look at nursing as a whole, it can be seen that nurses can be found both as victims and as offenders. When we call to mind the specific process women used to make a decision about their vocation, which relied on sacrificing one's own identity for the sake of self-sacrificial obedience, we can hardly be surprised at finding that most nurses accepted the new regime and remained convinced that they were only doing good. In this they were simultaneously both victim and offender. Imprisoned as they were in the professional ideal, nurses were able to be accomplices to murder without any personal feeling of guilt. Having given up responsibility for their own actions to a higher authority, they experienced themselves as victims once this authority no longer existed.

And so, after 1945, nursing, in common with nearly all other areas of society, is marked more by continuity than by new beginnings. As functionaries of the Nazi Party and all its subsidiaries, nurses' posts were taken away, but within a few years many had again assumed leadership roles. Due to the great need for nurses the process of 'de-nazification' could be speeded up.

In Germany, the main concern of the Allied Forces was to re-establish nursing services and nursing schools. There was a need to ensure care for survivors and for refugees, and so, by necessity, the professional knowledge of nurses was valued more highly than their tainted past. Many of the former Nazi nurses did not even destroy their brown uniform. They simply removed the stripes and the brooch and continued to work. The Allied Forces made great efforts in the early years to make fundamental changes in the foundations of nursing. However, finally the old 'tried and true' structures which had existed prior to 1933 reestablished themselves, and nurses remained bound to their traditions, at least with regard to what a new professionalism in all its consequences would have meant.

The way in which offenders were convicted in nursing was comparable to that of other professionals – a few were condemned to death, a number were sentenced to some years in prison and many were acquitted on the grounds that they had acted out of obedience and had killed only under orders. Most nurses who were accused of euthanasia continued to work as nurses after 1945, both before their sentences and after having served their time or being acquitted. To date, no case is known in which a nurse's right to practise was taken away because of participation in Nazi crimes.

CONCLUSION

In closing, I would like to offer some thoughts about what we can learn from history.

Nursing during National Socialism shows us how much the limits and possibilities of a profession are determined by a given society. Members of a profession are never only passive pawns on a chessboard, they are also active players. For nursing this might mean actively taking on this responsibility and trading in the dream of good, innocent nursing for reality. Nursing especially, has many decisions to make with regard to public health and therefore must be very clear what it can and cannot do from the point of view of the profession.

The history of our profession is not the history of sacrificing heroes and unstinting servers. Nurses were also weak, mediocre, despairing, competitive and scheming. They were betrayed and persecuted; they also fought back, they resisted and they learned from their mistakes. In short, they were quite normal people. The dark and the light sides of nursing are both part of what nursing means; only when we deal with both sides can nursing remain vital, honest and open, and develop further. The problem of inhumanity in health care is not confined to the time of National Socialism. As one of the professions concerned with public health services, nursing has the right and also the duty to treat humanely all who require nursing assistance. In order to be sensitive to all signs of inhumanity, it is necessary to confront any particular manifestation completely and uncompromisingly. German nursing especially has to accept responsibility for this part of its history. The crimes committed during National Socialism cannot be undone by keeping silent about them. Looking at them honestly can at least encourage reflection. And for millions of victims, keeping the memory alive is the only means of preventing this episode of history from being forgotten. Recent events in Germany show how important it is to confront the ideas and ideologies of extreme right-wing radicals. Nurses must also express their energetic opposition to any form of prejudice against foreigners. Confronting history in this way gives rise to many further questions which offer us opportunities for discussion and interchange. The way in which professions change under totalitarian regimes is not a uniquely German issue, but offers international nursing many opportunities for further research, reflection and comparative analysis.

It would perhaps be interesting to pose the question, worldwide, of the degree to which obedience and adaptation are still characteristic of good nursing, and how far we have really come with our demands for professional independence and self-determination.

NOTES

1 C. Bischoff, *Frauen in der Krankenpflege*, Frankfurt am Main, Campus, 1984

2 H-P. Schaper, *Krankenwartung und Krankenpflege*, Opladen, Leske und Budrich, 1987.

3 M. Rübenstahl, *Wilde Schwestern*, Frankfurt am Main, Mabuse, 1994.

4 H. Steppe (ed.), *Krankenpflege im Nationalsozialismus*, Frankfurt, Mabuse 1993, 7th edn, p. 33f.

5 G. Baader, 'Zur Ideologie des Sozialdarwinismus', in G. Baader and U. Schultz (eds), *Medizin und Nationalsozialismus*, Berlin, Verlagsgesellschaft Gesundheit, 1980, pp. 39–51.

6 S. Graessner, 'Gesundheitspolitik unterm Hakenkreuz', ibid., p. 145.

7 N. Frei (ed.), *Medizin und Gesundheitspolitik in der NS-Zeit*, München, Oldenbourg, 1991, p. 7.
8 ibid. In translating this slogan, the translator notes: 'It is difficult to capture the feeling or connotation associated with the words, phrases and slogans that had a specific meaning in the Nazi era. Even today Germans cannot use these words nor hear them without a shiver. The words are tainted with the whole history of the Third Reich.'
9 Archive material from the Head Office for Public Welfare, November 1936, contained in the German State's archives in Koblenz (Bundesarchives in Koblenz), (BA) R 36 1061 author's translation.
10 D. Reese and C. Sachse, 'Frauenforschung zum Nationalsozialismus', in L. Gravenhorst and C. Tatschmurat (eds), *Töchter-Fragen NS-Frauen-Geschichte*, Freiburg, Kore, 1990, pp. 73–106.
11 G. Bock, *Zwangssterilisation im Nationalsozialismus*, Opladen, Westdeutscher Verlag, 1986, p. 133.
12 B. Braun, 'Die Frauenbewegung am Scheidewege', special printing from *Weltkampf*, 1932, p. 8 (Bundesarchives (BA), N.S.D., 47/14 author's translation).
13 G. Scholtz-Klink, 'Kundgebung aller schaffenden Frauen', in *Zeitschrift der Reichsfachschaft Deutscher Schwestern und Pflegerinnen*, 26 October 1934, vol. 2, no. 11, p. 226 author's translation.
14 Advertising brochure, 1938, Bundesarchives (BA): R36 881 author's translation.
15 E. Mach, 'NSV-Schwesternschaft', in *Zeitschrift der Reichsfachschaft Deutscher Schwestern und Pflegerinnen*, 1934, vol. 2, no. 3, pp. 44–45 (author's translation).
16 Advertising brochure, 1938, Bundesarchives (BA): R36 881 author's translation.
17 H. Jensen, 'Sinn, Zweck und Ziel der NS-Schwesternschaft', special printing from *Zeitschrift der Reichsfachschaft Deutscher Schwestern und Pflegerinnen*, Berlin, Elwin Staude, 1934, vol. 2, no. 8, p. 4f. author's translation.
18 H. Vorländer, *Die NSV, Darstellung und Dokumentation einer Nationalsozialistischen Organisation*, Boppard, Harald Boldt, 1988, p. 6ff. author's translation.
19 Bundesarchives (BA), Koblenz, NS 37 1039 (author's translation).
20 Steppe, op. cit., p. 53 author's translation.
21 Quoted in Steppe, op. cit., p. 9.
22 Quoted in Steppe, op. cit., p. 107.
23 Quoted in Steppe, op. cit., p. 9.
24 L. Katscher, *Krankenpflege und 'Drittes Reich'. Der Weg der Schwesternschaft des Evangelischen Diakonievereins*, Stuttgart, Verlagswerk der Diakonie, 1990, p. 83.
25 Prozessakten (case files), Strafsache gegen Erdmann u.a. (legal proceedings against Erdmann et al.), Bayrisches Staatsarchive (archives of the State of Bavaria), reference: 112 Ks 2/64, p. 333 author's translation.
26 ibid., p. 347.
27 Prozessakten (case files), Strafsache gegen Erdmann u.a. (legal pro-

ceedings against Erdmann *et al.*), op. cit., testimony of Gerda S., p. 537.
28 Prozessakten (case files), Strafsache gegen Erdmann u.a. (legal proceedings against Erdmann *et al.*), op. cit., testimony of Margarete T., p. 763.
29 Prozessakten (case files), Strafsache gegen Erdmann u.a. (legal proceedings against Erdmann *et al.*), op. cit., testimony of Luise E., p. 367.
30 R. Weglein, *Als Krankenschwester im KZ Thereisienstadt*, Stuttgart, Silberburg, 1988, p. 44.

Chapter 2

The legacy of the history of nursing for post-apartheid South Africa

Shula Marks

In September 1995 South Africa's public sector hospitals were in turmoil as black nurses went on strike and took to the streets. Newspaper headlines alleged that patients were dying for lack of care, and front-page pictures showed harassed junior doctors working marathon hours.[1] 'Florence Nightingale died at Baragwanath this week' proclaimed one usually thoughtful observer of the health scene.[2]

The strike aroused particular anguish, for at the heart of post-apartheid South Africa's plans for transforming its health services are the country's approximately 165,000 registered and enrolled nurses, enrolled nursing auxiliaries and student nurses.[3] Of these probably about one third are white, the rest African, Coloured and Asian.[4] In large parts of the Republic, especially in the rural areas, health care is in the hands of black nurses, with only very occasional visits from a medical practitioner.[5] Recent changes in the law allowing nurses to act as diagnosticians and dispense drugs recognize their *de facto* position as the main purveyors of health care to the African populace. Over 95 per cent of these nurses are women, and, although in the last decade an increasing number have moved into the private sector, the majority of African nurses are probably still in state employment.[6] Among Africans, fully qualified, registered nurses outnumber the entire male professional and semi-professional elite, and there can be little doubt that nurses – of all ranks – are an invaluable source of skilled person-power.

Yet, as the 1995 strike revealed, the profession is divided and embattled as never before, excoriated in the press and palpably demoralized. There was, it is true, a certain historical amnesia about the media coverage. Black nurses' strikes from the 1980s onwards had been met with almost identical banner headlines and photographs. In recent years, stories of the 'bad nurse' have become a recurrent theme in popular discourses – in the newspapers and among doctors and administrators as well as among the lay public; the narratives appear to weave together nineteenth-century Dickensian images of 'Sairey Gamp' with African rumours of nursing cruelty.[7] There were, of course, specific reasons for the eruption of anger by the nurses and the form it took in August 1995. Yet the anger was neither new nor unpredictable.

Over the last decade, at least, nursing in South Africa has faced a crisis of major proportions, one which it shares with the profession internationally, but which has its own particularities.[8] Everywhere, transformations in the health care system and escalating health care costs, together with the consequent shift in the locus of decision-making to a new managerial bureaucracy, as well as changing social expectations and political values, have contributed to an intense debate about the profession's future. This forms part of a wide-ranging questioning of its historic values and is closely related to the equally wide questioning of the legitimacy of the hospital and high technology heath care.

Many of these trends have been evident also in South Africa, but if, by 1990, nurses internationally had reached a 'crossroads', nurses in South Africa have been in the eye of the storm.[9] Not only have they experienced many of the broader international trends affecting the health care system as a whole; many were drawn into the turbulent politics of South Africa, not least because of the history of the profession and the state's own politicization of health care in general and nursing in particular over the past forty years. Above all, they faced the legacy of a health care system which, by the early 1990s, was itself in severe crisis, the result of the concentration of health workers in 'sophisticated curative settings' and private clinics in urban, middle-class, white areas and their scarcity in the largely black rural and peri-urban areas, informal settlements; the inappropriate training and professionalism of many health workers; and the fragmentation of the health services.[10] Appalling conditions in many public and teaching hospitals had hit the newspaper headlines over the previous decade and more.

The inheritance of the past weighs heavily on post-apartheid health policy, and both the divisions within the South African nursing profession and its demoralization can be traced to the complex legacy of its history.[11] Professional nursing in South Africa traces its origins to English 'lady nurses' on the Nightingale model, drawn from the Anglican (and, to a lesser extent, Roman Catholic) sisterhoods. In its early days, the nursing profession in South Africa reflected the gender/class divisions as well as the internal hierarchies which characterized the profession in nineteenth-century Britain. These meshed well not only with the patriarchal structure of colonial society but also with its racial and ethnic structures.

Class attitudes brought to South Africa by the English 'lady nurses' were rapidly transmuted into racial attitudes, and became even more important in the confused and ambiguous world of the colonial hospital, a world where noble aspirations and polluting domestic labour constantly rubbed shoulders, and where domestic labour was not only associated with the lower classes but also with the 'inferior races'. Class and race boundaries had to be jealously preserved and were marked out on the body in the shape of uniform, badge and insignia, in the rigid hierarchies and careful delineation of roles and status and in the innumerable rules regulating every aspect of behaviour.

So long as nursing remained in the hands of the celibate and asexual Anglican and Catholic sisterhoods, which founded professional nursing in the region, colonial apprehensions around issues of black sexuality and racial pollution were not too pronounced. However, by the turn of the century, not all nurses were drawn from the sisterhoods: working- or lower-class English women, many of whom had come out to nurse during the South African war, had joined the profession and a chorus of voices demanded an end to white nursing of black male patients. It was at least in part in response to these white racial anxieties that non-conformist missionaries took up the challenge to train black women as registered nurses. Drawn from the educated elite, many of them third-generation Christians, the first black registered nurses were, in the words of the African writer, H.I.E. Dhlomo, 'Bantu Nightingales'.[12]

From the earliest days, the missionaries deliberately inculcated western values which served to distance the nurses from their communities, and create a new middle-class elite. Their entire education from mission school to nursing college was designed to give them a new identity which was far removed from the 'ignorance' and 'superstition', the 'barbarity' and 'bestiality' of native life. They were to moralize and save, not simply to nurse, the sick.[13] The discourse of western scientific medicine and the missionaries have remarkable continuities. For Charlotte Searle, the doyen of South African nursing for almost half a century from the 1940s, as for the missionary doctors who trained the first black nurses, 'Scientific medicine had . . . to conquer witchcraft and nursing [was] its standard bearer'.[14] This ethos has powerfully mediated the relationship between nurses and their patients.

Ironically, professional nursing, the most prestigious occupation for African women in twentieth-century South Africa, had its origins in late nineteenth–early twentieth-century anxieties around notions of racial purity. Yet the racial boundaries thus established in the very origins of black nursing always sat uncomfortably with the universalist discourse of the health professional. This fundamental tension in the relationship between white doctors and nurses and black patients set up profound ambiguities for the healing professions. Racist medical practice was frequently at odds with a liberal ideology which demanded of the doctor and nurse that they provide health care 'regardless of race, colour or creed', and which placed a premium on a single professional standard for the state's recognition of the nurse's status.[15]

These ideals came under even greater strain in the inter-war years, when (white) Afrikaner women were recruited into the profession in large numbers for the first time, to reach 70 per cent of the total by the mid-century. In the 1930s and 1940s they provided a highly exploited workforce in the hospitals, and were treated with disdain and condescension by the English lady-nurses who controlled the upper echelons of the profession. The tensions were explosive, and the junior Afrikaner nurses were readily mobilizable either by Afrikaner nationalists (as they were in the 1950s) or by the trade union movement (a familiar phenomenon internationally and one which had later parallels among junior black nurses).

Indeed it was their fear of the 'menace of trade unionism' which led the South African state to agree to the demands from nursing leaders for a 'closed shop' Nursing Association and an autonomous Nursing Council independent of the Medical Council in 1944, something both the state and the doctors had strenuously

resisted only five years before as 'quite premature'. The hostility
of the nursing leaders to trade unionism, and the particular
alliance they forged with the state in their struggle to achieve
control in the 1944 Nursing Act, shaped the profession over the
next half-century. The failure of the Nursing Association to
achieve effective negotiating machinery at this time lay partly
behind the chronically low wage structure of the profession, and
has contributed to the turbulence of recent times.

At the same time, the growing concordat between the Nursing
Council and the state from the mid-century seriously comprom-
ised its leadership in the eyes of black nurses, and remained a
serious source of tension even after the dramatic changes of the
1990s. If in the 1940s many Afrikaans-speaking nurses had felt
dominated from above by English 'lady-nurses', many also felt
threatened from below by the as-yet small, but growing, class of
highly qualified professional black nurses, who were trained
mainly in the mission hospitals, but who passed the same examin-
ations and achieved the same qualifications as their white counterparts. And whereas the small number of African registered nurses
was drawn from the middle-class elite, the majority of Afrikaner
women came from working-class and rural backgrounds so that
their racial and class identities and assumptions were at odds with
one another. This led to the strident calls for the segregation of
the profession, especially after the Afrikaner National Party
won the 1948 election, and a section of white nurses were mobili-
zed for the apartheid cause.

Internationally, one of the dominant themes in the history of
nursing is the fundamental tension between the insistence of its
leaders that nursing is a profession for refined and educated
middle-class women, and the amount of domestic labour
demanded by the occupation. In South Africa this was further
complicated by the widespread association of cleaning and scrubbing – a major part of the nurse's duties at least until the mid-
twentieth century – with black rather than white hands. Thus, the
drive towards professionalization, so central a characteristic of
the history of nursing in Britain and the United States of
America, had in South Africa both a class and an urgent racial
agenda.

If nursing was to be a respectable occupation for white women,
the stigma of domestic labour had to be removed; and control
over the profession had to be kept white. This was even more

important in view of the ambiguous relationship between the race and class of the black and white nurses, and fuelled both the establishment of academic nursing departments and the demands for legislation to segregate the hitherto non-racial Nursing Association and Council. Vigorously contested both within South Africa and without, the Nursing Amendment Act of 1957 – at one level an outcome of the racialized pursuit of professionalism by white nurses – was to lead to their forced withdrawal from the International Council of Nurses. This was a bitter blow to their professional identity, and one which was to contribute to the reform of apartheid in nursing from the late 1980s.

Paradoxically however, it was under apartheid after 1948, when the profession was most effectively legally segregated, that the numbers of African nurses expanded dramatically, and the racial barriers collapsed under the dire shortage of white nurses. By the 1950s, with the intensification of black urbanization and industrialization, the provision of health care in the major urban centres became an urgent necessity for the reproduction of the black working class, however inadequate that provision may have been. And the racial ideology of the state dictated that patients be cared for only by nurses of the same race. That the highly-paid doctors remained for the most part white, regardless of the skin-colour of their patients, seems to have escaped the notice of the racial ideologues. (Maleness – or the status of doctor – apparently provided protection against pollution by racial contact.)

Increasingly, however, nursing – even beyond the confines of the black hospitals – became a black profession, albeit one dominated by a largely Afrikanerized female bureaucracy, prepared to accommodate to apartheid ideology. The increase in numbers, from some 800 fully registered black nurses in 1948 to about 100,000 in 1990, is remarkable. It was accompanied by increasing numbers of black nurses in senior and specialized posts. Black nurses also became subject to the same processes of professionalization established in the 1950s for Afrikaner women, through the constant raising of entrance qualifications and the attachment of nursing to the universities. As elsewhere, however, this process did not solve the acute shortage of nurses in the public hospitals, and it has exacerbated old divisions and created fresh ones within the black sisterhood in the early 1990s.

To understand the contemporary crisis in health care and current divisions in the profession, it is necessary not only to take account of this general historical background, but also to rehearse briefly the challenges which have confronted the South African state since 1970. Over this period, population increase, together with the continued displacement of Africans from white agriculture and the intensified impoverishment and political oppression in the so-called African 'homelands', accelerated African urbanization and rendered the pass laws inoperable. The country's political geography was transformed as influx controls were abandoned and ever larger numbers of desperate Africans poured into the cities, and huge squatter areas grew up in their environs. The weaknesses of the apartheid economy were increasingly manifest, and were exacerbated by international sanctions and the low-intensity war South Africa waged against her newly independent neighbours. Economic recession and high levels of unemployment – estimated at between 40 and 70 per cent of the workforce by 1990 – has meant that increasing numbers of people even in the urban areas are without proper nutrition, clean water, adequate sewerage or decent housing, while by the end of the 1980s AIDS loomed as a new, if as yet only partially realized, threat.[16]

Internally, African opposition stepped up and by the mid-1980s had erupted in urban insurrection. State attempts to defuse African protest through welfare fragmented the once monolithic National Party and politicized black civil society to an unprecedented degree. Finally in February 1990 the banned liberation organizations were unbanned and the imprisoned leader of the African National Congress (ANC), Nelson Mandela, was released. The era ended with the elections at the end of April 1994, and the formation of a transitional government in which the ANC was the dominant partner.

As political turmoil and economic deprivation mounted, nurses across the country were caught up in the frontline of the consequent violence, as ordinary members of the public, as mothers, wives, sisters and daughters, but also as carers who had to tend bruised, bleeding and battered bodies and bury the dead. Caught between their duties to their patients and the demands of the comrades, between the pressures of the community and the discipline of the Nursing Council, many found themselves facing conflicting demands from new radical health organizations and unions on the one hand and their professional association, the Nursing Council and the state, on the other. By the early 1990s, nurses could be threatened with death for going on strike – and threatened with death for not going on strike.[17]

As an anonymous matron at the time of a strike at the Baragwanath Hospital in 1992 put it, nurses

> are intimidated from all sides from the strikers who see us as scabs, from our bosses who threaten to fire us, from our own disciplinary body, the South African Nursing Council (SANC) which [now] tells us that we have the right to strike, but which also tells us that if we leave our patients to spend even an hour on the picket-line we will be struck off the roll.[18]

It should also be remembered that all this was being played out against broader changes in the health care system. As in other parts of the world, so in South Africa, there was a shift in the government's view of the relationship of the private to the public sector in the 1980s. The worldwide move to monetarist policies saw an equally widespread call for the reordering of health priorities towards more effective and lower-cost medical strategies. High-technology medical care, introduced since the 1950s, was now seen as too expensive even for developed countries, and was demonstrably inappropriate for developing ones. This led to the advocacy of two different types of solution, privatization for the more affluent in the western industrialized countries, and primary health care for the poor in the Third World.

In line with its conceit that the Republic combined the problems of the First and the Third World, the South African government appropriated the rhetoric of both the privatization and the primary health care lobbies.[19] Given its contradictory and high-cost policies of fragmenting health services, and its desire to create and co-opt the black middle class, the government increasingly looked to the private sector to make health care provision not only for whites but also for more affluent blacks – including nurses in the public hospitals – through private health insurance schemes. By the end of the decade, in the face of one of the worst recessions in South Africa's history, this drive was accelerated as the government desperately attempted to reduce public expenditure.[20]

At the same time, throughout the 1980s much lip-service was paid to primary health care especially in the rural and black urban areas. Yet its actual practice remained patchy and ambiguous.[21] For most of the decade the large provincial tertiary hospitals continued to absorb between 70 and 80 per cent of the health budget; less than 5 per cent went to preventive medicine, and primary and community health care remained underdeveloped.[22]

Whatever the shifts in policy, there was an ever greater demand for better-trained nurses – to take charge of the new primary health care centres, to work in the public hospitals and to provide the personnel for the largely white private health care facilities. And while, as we have seen, nursing numbers were indeed expanded, an increasing number of these were now in the private sector.[23] Thus by the beginning of 1990 the South African Nursing Association was warning of the imminent collapse of the public sector under multiple demands.[24] Part of this was a familiar problem: the public sector found it difficult to compete with the private sector in the recruitment of staff, given a disparity in salaries, more night duty, higher patient–staff ratios, and deteriorating conditions in the chronically overcrowded, and still segregated, black wards.[25] In the black hospitals, appalling overcrowding and the shortage of basic materials inevitably demoralized and alienated nursing staff. Not surprisingly, increasing numbers of doctors and nurses, including black nurses, were drawn into the predominantly white private sector.[26]

Although it was heralded as the solution to some of the health sector's problems, the further professionalization of nurses' education in the 1980s did little to alleviate the crisis. In 1983, in line with international developments, colleges of nursing became part of the tertiary education system for the first time and in 1986 their association with university nursing departments became obligatory.[27] In that year, too, the Nursing Council increased the training for the general registered nurse from three to four years. General nursing and midwifery, as well as psychiatry and community health, which had previously been post-basic courses, were now included in an integrated syllabus.

In justifying the move to university attachment and in deploring the ratio of enrolled to fully qualified nurses, South Africa's nursing leaders couched their arguments in the familiar language of international nursing.[28] The attachment to the tertiary sector and the new integrated four-year degree would educate the more autonomous nurse needed for primary or community health care, and provide the high level of training needed for increasingly demanding jobs. Like liberal feminist writers on nursing internationally they stressed the importance of the shift in nurses' training from apprenticeship in the wards to college-based education in expanding opportunities for women. The need for a more flexible and open-ended education in the face of new developments in society and medicine is widely acknowledged.[29]

Yet, as elsewhere, the pursuit of professionalism through the university sector has not changed the power relations in the health sector. As Celia Davies has remarked more widely in discussing the predicament of contemporary nursing: 'Nursing is still an adjunct to a gendered concept of profession. Nursing is the activity ... that enables medicine to present itself as masculine/ rational and to gather the power and privilege of doing so.'[30] University training merely heightens the predicament because it is premised on the same qualities. Nor does it challenge the subordination of nurses to doctors or the internal hierarchy of the nursing profession, with its historical divisions between black and white, junior and senior, registered, enrolled and auxiliary nurses. On the contrary, it adds a further distinction between the university- and the college-trained nurse.

Thus, at the same time as a small number of nurses became increasingly specialized, acquiring new, better-rewarded skills, the majority were reduced to the more menial tasks, working long hours in overcrowded wards, subordinate within a rigidly organized nursing hierarchy, and with little control over their working lives.[31] Already in the 1950s the matron of Baragwanath Hospital talked of the 'rapidly changing pattern' of nursing, especially in large, city hospitals, where the turnover of patients was so much more rapid.[32] Thirty years later, according to Rispel and Schneider, nursing, in the large hospitals, had

> become more like a production line in a factory, where ... each nurse is assigned to tasks such as bed-making, backwashing, or distribution of medication. ... There is little time for bedside work, family contact, and personal involvement in the recovery of patients.[33]

Thus 'while nursing has become increasingly sophisticated in its theory and training, the working experience of many nurses has actually involved an erosion of control and autonomy'.[34]

This is true also of nurses' experience of the new training outside of the small numbers (well under 10 per cent) who get a university place. Inherited from the history of the profession is a rigid and authoritarian form of education.[35] Despite the attachment of nursing colleges to the university sector, much nursing education remains by rote, encouraging conformity rather than innovation. Even now, many nurses find during their training that 'it is much better not to question or comment on what happens either in nursing college or in hospital wards'. Their socialization 'creates a fear of victimisation, an unquestioning attitude and a strong feeling that anonymous conformity is safe'.[36] While university affiliation may redress this in time, actual practice still lags behind the rhetoric of nursing leaders.[37]

If anything, the pursuit of professionalism and the new managerialism in nursing may have exacerbated the crisis in nursing in South Africa as it has elsewhere, perhaps because, as Celia Davies has recently argued, the very concept of professionalism is not gender-neutral and is dictated by a series of what she terms masculine qualities and norms, which in themselves pose problems for women in nursing.[38] Nor does the pursuit of professionalism address the paucity of educated women willing to fill the qualified nursing role.[39]

The debate about professionalization is crucial to the future of nursing in South Africa. The debate is the familiar one between those who wish to see nursing as a profession for well-educated, largely middle-class women, and those who see the urgent need for more hands-on and primary health carers at lower cost. In the South African case even more than the British one, an elitist professional model of nursing care pays scant attention to economic realities and has little hope of serving the needs of the majority of the people. The deeply entrenched ideology of professionalism and the emphasis on status, as well as the middle-class aspirations of the fully trained nurses frequently creates a gulf between such nurses and their patients, as well as between the fully trained and the enrolled categories and other hospital staff.[40]

As elsewhere, societal change, and especially new expectations on the part of women, have increased nurses' dissatisfaction with conditions which earlier generations were prepared to tolerate. Nurses no longer remain within the tightly controlled confines of the nurses' home throughout their training, and the old sense of duty and obligation regardless of material well-being has been undermined. They are no longer so willing to accept the long hours, poor pay and backbreaking work as inevitable. White nurses have voted with their feet and simply moved out of the profession; many (though by no means a majority of) African nurses, with fewer economic alternatives, and in a general context of black political radicalization, have looked for remedies beyond what appear to be the ineffectual negotiations of the Nursing Association or even, more recently, the activities of the trade unions which they identify with the needs of the non-professional health workers.[41]

Unfortunately neither decrees from the Ministry of Health nor the undoubted changes within the South African Nursing Association and the South African Nursing Council which have taken place over the past few years can transform the legacies of history overnight. The dualisms in South Africa's health services – between primary health care for the poor and private health care for the better off; between superior doctors and inferior nurses; between a powerful professional elite and a powerless majority of less qualified carers – continue to bedevil the profession, as do the gendered stereotypes associated with these dualisms, as some nursing leaders attempt to find an identity for the embattled profession through a return to the concept of 'caring' as a specific female attribute, as opposed to the 'male' 'academic' model of the nurse practitioner.

The vision of nursing as a quintessentially female domain, distinguished from the 'male' medical model by its practice of the 'womanly' virtues of caring and compassion, dies hard at top levels of the profession, despite the fact that women constitute an increasingly large proportion of medical students, and despite the harsh realities of contemporary hospital nursing.[42] Yet this notion simply perpetuates many of the problems which have haunted nursing since its inception, when the acceptance of 'the contemporary assumption that there was a necessary and laudable conjunction between nursing and femininity' and that 'the trained sensibility of a middle-class woman could alone bring order and morality to the hospital's grim wards' incorporated attitudes towards gender and class that were to contribute to the chronic problems of nursing as an underpaid profession dependent on the sense of self-sacrifice of women.[43]

As recent writers on nursing have begun to stress, until health systems are rethought as a whole, and the relationships between care and cure, community and clinic, doctor and nurse, patient and 'professional', are transformed, the more flexible and empowering modalities needed for primary and community health care will remain as elusive as ever.

NOTES

1 See, for example, *The Star* (Johannesburg), 6 Sept. 1995, for both the headline and the picture.

2 Pat Sidley in *Weekly Mail and Guardian*, 8–14 Sept. 1995, vol. 11, no. 37, pp. 6–7. The article was headlined, 'Florence Nightingale turns in her grave'.

3 For the role of nurses as '*frontline providers* of clinical PHC services' and more generally for the importance of PHC in the government's health plans, see *Restructuring the National Health System for Universal Primary Health Care. Report of the Committee of Inquiry into a National Health Insurance System*, Pretoria, Department of Health, 1995, 3 vols. The italics are in the orginal phrase, in vol. I, *Executive Summary*, p. S.6.

4 These figures can only be approximate. According to the South African Nursing Council, at the end of 1994 there were some 159,000 nurses on their rolls, of whom about 5,000 were working outside South Africa; they estimated that there were a further 25,000 on the rolls of the former Transkei, Bophuthatswana, Venda and Ciskei Nursing Councils, but about half of these with dual registration. There were in addition over 15,500 student and pupil nurses, whom I have included in the total in the text, as they provide a crucial component of the hospital labour-force. Since the early 1990s the Nursing Council has not classified nurses on its registers by race, but the proportional breakdown has probably not changed much since then. In 1990 just under one-third of the nurses were white, but over two-thirds of them were qualified; only 40 per cent of the African nurses, the vast majority of the black nurses, had the full four-year qualification. (See SAIRR, *Survey of Race Relations 1991/2*, Johannesburg, 1992, pp. 121–2; and C. Searle, 'South Africa celebrates 100 years of state registration of nurses and midwives 1891–1991', *Nursing RSA Verpleging*, 1991, vol. 6, no. 3, p. 8.)

I am grateful to Mr Allan Green at SANC for providing the statistics and explaining some of the complexities of the nursing statistics to me (interview, 14 September 1995).

5 I use the term 'black' to refer to Indians, Coloureds and Africans. South African state terminology refers only to Africans as 'blacks'.

6 See R. Thompson, 'The development of nursing', in R. White (ed.), *Issues in Nursing: Past, Present and Future*, Chichester, John Wiley & Sons, 1988, p. 180, and L.R. Uys, 'Racism and the South African nurse', *Nursing RSA Verpleging*, Nov.–Dec. 1987, vol. 2, nos. 11/12, p. 55.

7 For this widespread image in the media, see D. Keet, 'Organising in the health sector: nurses', *SALB*, 1992, vol. 16, no. 7, pp. 51–5; for similar views expressed by a Groote Schuur nurse ten years earlier,

see C. Stern, 'The love-hate battle of the nursing profession', *Cape Times*, 22 Aug. 1981. M. Resha, *'Mangoana O Toara Thipa Ka Bohaleng*, London and Johannesburg, Congress of South African Writers, 1991, p. 21; and B.A. Pauw, *The Second Generation*, 2nd edn, Cape Town, London and New York, 1973, pp. 81–2, suggest the image has longer roots. I was regaled with similar reports in the late 1980s/early 1990s.

8 *Verpleging/Nursing RSA*, 1990, vol. 5, no. 4, p. 6; P. Owens and H. Glennirster, *Nursing in Conflict*, Basingstoke, Macmillan Education, 1990, pp. 19, 29; C. Rosenberg, *Explaining Epidemics and Other Studies in the History of Medicine*, New York, Cambridge University Press, 1992, Chapter 16.

9 The term is from Owens and Glennerster, op. cit., p. 19.

10 See, for example, African National Congress, *A National Health Plan for South Africa*, Johannesburg, 1994, p. 32.

11 I have dealt with this history in detail in: S Marks, *Divided Sisterhood. Race, Class and Gender in the South African Nursing Profession*, Basingstoke and Johannesburg, Macmillan, 1994, which also provides the references for what follows.

12 In a poem in his unpublished play *Malaria*.

13 See Chapter 4, in Marks, op. cit., and A.P. Cheater, 'A marginal elite? A study of African registered nurses in the Greater Durban area', MA dissertation, 1972, University of Natal, Durban. As late as 1967, Dr H.H. Stott of the Valley Trust, a non-governmental community project aimed at eliminating malnutrition, inveighed against the 'ignorance and superstition' of the 'Bantu attitude to illness' in an address to African nurses. 'With this background', he continued, 'it is not surprising that the average Bantu selects his food for no other consideration than for filling qualities and palatability' ('The Valley Trust', *SANJ*, July 1967, pp. 24–5).

14 'Professional advancement of the African nurse', *SANJ*, Feb. 1961, p. 28; see also her 'South African nursing credo', South African Nursing Association, Pretoria, 1980, which emphasizes the religious foundation of nursing.

15 Ibid., p. 612.

16 S.M. Benatar, 'Medicine and health care in South Africa – five years later', *New England Journal of Medicine*, 4 July 1991, vol. 325, no. 1, p. 16. For the deterioration in health status, see Department of National Health and Population Development, *1990 Health Trends*, Pretoria, 1991, which showed *inter alia* increased malnutrition rates for Coloureds, Indians and Whites; an increase in the number of TB cases among Africans of 22 per cent and among Coloureds of 35 per cent between 1986 and 1989, increased notification rates of hepatitis for all sectors of the population, and rapidly increasing rates of HIV infection. In general the evidence from South Africa is extremely difficult to read, not least because of the exclusion of the 'homelands' from the pre-1994 official statistics, and the absence of any national registration of births and deaths for Africans.

17 This paragraph is based on newspaper cuttings (see, for example,

'Striking nurses at Umlazi hospital receive death threats', *Daily News*, 6 Sept. 1991), and interviews with Matron Bolanyi, McCord Hospital, Durban, 29 July 1988; a group of nurses in Soweto in Aug. 1989 who wished to remain anonymous; a matron in the Ciskei, 27 July 1989, who wished to remain anonymous; a visit to the Jane Furse Hospital, in July 1988, and interviews with Mrs van der Walt and others, Groote Schuur, 11 Sept. 1992, and with Noel Hunt and Heidi Brookes, 21 Sept. 1992. The widespread intimidation of nurses sometimes made it difficult to conduct interviews.

18 M. Gevisser, 'Behind the barricades', *Weekly Mail*, 17 to 23 July 1992.

19 Department of Health and Welfare, *National Plan for Health Service Facilities*, Pretoria, 1980, p. 7.

20 See, for example, S.M. Benatar, 'Medicine and health care in South Africa'; 'Report from Parliament', in *Nursing RSA Verpleging* 1990, vol. 5, no. 4, p. 5; Fred Krockott, 'The nightmare when nurses go on strike' and 'Run-down Edendale expected to precipitate a crisis', in *Sunday Tribune*, 9 Sept. 1991.

21 The most imaginative primary health care took place outside of the state sector, and was undertaken in the main by non-governmental agencies.

22 See, for example, D. Yach *et al.*, *Changing Health in South Africa. Towards New Perspectives*, Henry J. Kaiser Foundation, Menlo Park, California, 1991, pp. 36–7.

23 For the increased numbers see references in note 4 above. M. Zwarenstein has estimated that by 1990–1, 60 per cent of all nurses were in the private sector; the percentage of black nurses in private practice would probably be lower (cited in Yach *et al.* op. cit., p. 43).

24 See references in note 20 above.

25 According to Harry Schwartz, Democratic Party spokesman on finance, in 1990, 49 per cent of beds reserved for whites in the public hospitals were empty (*Nursing RSA Verpleging*, 1990, vol. 5, no. 4, in the parliamentary debate on the Additional Appropriation Bill). In May 1990 the Minister for Health announced the end of segregation in hospitals; nevertheless, in 1991 there were still 22 all-white provincial hospitals, mostly in the Orange Free State and Transvaal (SAIRR, *Race Relations Survey, 1991/2*, pp. 124–7).

26 Benatar, op. cit., p. 31. *Survey of Race Relations 1991/2*, p. 122.

27 R. Thompson, op. cit., p. 179. Note that this was in advance of proposals of the UK Central Council for Nursing, Midwifery and Health Visiting (UKCC) *Project 2000: a new preparation for practice*, London, UKCC, 1986.

28 Searle discusses this at some length in *Towards Excellence. The centenary of state registration for nurses and midwives in South Africa, 1891–1991*, Durban, Butterworths 1991, pp. 260–1.

29 See, for example, B. Melosh, *The Physician's Hand: work, culture and conflict in American nursing*, Philadelphia, 1982, pp. 70 ff; and for a recent British statement, UKCC, op. cit.

30 C. Davies, *Gender and the Professional Predicament in Nursing*, Milton Keynes, Open University Press, 1995.

31 See, for example, Stern, op. cit.
32 University of Witwatersrand, A2197. B1.4 Jane McLarty Papers, Study Course in African culture and its relationship to the training of African nurses, Nov. 1954, 'Summary and assessment' by Jane McLarty.
33 L. Rispel and H. Schneider, 'Professionalization of South African nursing: who benefits?', in L. Rispel (ed.), *Nursing at the Crossroads: Organisation, Professionalisation and Politicisation*, symposium proceedings, published by the Centre for the Study of Health Policy, University of Witwatersrand, 1990, pp. 111–12.
34 Ibid., pp. 111–12.
35 See, for example, B. Robertson, J.K. Large, N. Selebano *et al.*, 'An evaluation of the Specialist Nurse Practitioner', *SAMJ*, Nov. 1979, vol. 56, no. 17: 'Training in the clinical subjects was rigid and regimented. . . . Each subject was assigned to one person, or at most two. . . . This ensured uniformity, facilitated indoctrination and eliminated irrelevant differences of opinion. Diverse opinions would confuse the students and defeat the objective of simplicity' (pp. 836–7). This was the philosophy advocated for a post-basic training programme for 'specialist nurses' in primary care settings by a group of senior black and white nurses and a black physician.
36 L. Rispel and M. Motsei, 'Nursing in South Africa: exploring nurses' opinions on controversial issues', Centre for the Study of Health Policy, University of Witwatersrand, n.d. (paper presented to the ASSA conference Durban, 1988).
37 This at least appeared to be the consensus of nurses at the University of Cape Town seminar I addressed in Apr. 1991. While the university teachers present maintained that these practices were now a matter of the past, the college students were vociferous that they were not.
38 C. Davies, 1994, op. cit.
39 Owens and Glennerster, op. cit., p. 33. R. Dingwall, A.M. Rafferty and C. Webster, *An Introduction to the Social History of Nursing*, London, Routledge, 1988, pp. 206–7, and pp. 223–8 make this point in relation to British nursing; in South Africa as new opportunities open up for educated black women, it is becoming ever more important.
40 For a pertinent statement of this, see Clive Evian, 'The Tintswalo Hospital Primary Health Care Nurse Training Programme' in C.P. Owen and E.M. Thomson, *People's Health – The Way Forward. Report of the 1988 Namda Annual Conference*, Namda, Durban, 1991, pp. 55–6.
41 Part of the background to the Aug. 1995 strike was the large rise gained by the National Educational and Health Workers' Union for the poorest paid health workers, which eroded differentials, and led to the highly unusual sight of senior nurses going on strike, leaving students to run the wards.
42 Of South African medical students, 40 per cent were female in 1988 (Editorial, 'Nursing in the RSA', *SAMJ*, 18 Nov. 1989, vol. 76, p. 526). The sentence is based more broadly on oral evidence provided

during seminars held in the Department of Community Health and the African Studies Centre, both at the University of Cape Town, in Mar.–Apr. 1991.

43 C. Rosenberg, *The Care of Strangers; The Rise of America's Hospital System*, New York, Basic Books, 1987.

Chapter 3

The Rockefeller Agenda for American/Philippines nursing relations[1]

Barbara L. Brush

The Philippines leads all countries in global nurse emigration. Today, Filipino nurses represent over 75 per cent of the foreign nurse labour force recruited to and working in American hospitals, most of which are inner-city municipally operated institutions with reported shortages of nursing personnel. This article examines the historical roots of the American/Philippines nursing relationship more generally and the particular role of the Rockefeller Foundation in the 20th-century emigration patterns and work practices of Filipino nurses. Examination of one group of nurse workers enhances an understanding of the ways in which social, cultural, economic, and political factors influence broader health care decisions.

Between 1945 and 1990, thousands of nurses migrated to the United States to either learn or work in American hospitals. Most of the nurses in the first two decades after the second World War were participants in the Exchange Visitor Program (EVP), established through the International Council of Nurses (ICN) in 1948 (Brush, 1993). After 1965, the majority of nurse emigrants were recruited directly to United States hospitals for employment purposes. This shift was due in part to the combined effects of new and more liberal American immigration policies, greater consumer access to health care services, scepticism about EVP practices, hospital expansion, and a perception among hospitals and policymakers of the need for more nurses (Brush, 1994).

In addition to foreign nurses' changing status was a marked shift in their countries of origin. The almost exclusive European exchange visitor of the 1950s became the Asian nurse employee by the 1960s. For example, while Danish (14 per cent), Norwegian

(6 per cent), British (9 per cent), and Swedish (11 per cent) nurses represented the largest number of nurse migrants to the United States immediately after World War II (American Nurses' Association, 1951), Filipino nurses comprised 43 per cent of the American foreign nurse labour market by 1970. By the mid-1980s, these trends would continue; nurses from the Philippines represented 75 per cent of the total foreign nurse pool working in United States hospitals.

To date, the Philippines continues to lead all other countries in global nurse emigration. In 1989, an estimated 13,000 new nurses graduated from 132 nursing schools in the Philippines, 65 per cent of whom emigrated abroad, and many to American hospitals (Gonzales, 1989). Most of these institutions, according to a report by the United States General Accounting Office (1989), were inner-city, municipally operated hospitals with reported shortages of nursing personnel.

Although foreign nurses comprise only 4 per cent of the total American nursing workforce, their presence in many geographically situated hospitals across the nation is often critical to institutions' continued operations. Nonetheless, foreign nurses have often been ignored in discussions of nurse manpower development more generally. The aims of this article are to examine Filipino nurses as one particular group of foreign nurses as a means to answer several broader questions. Why do Filipino nurses emigrate in such large numbers, and why are they the preferred or, at least, most commonly employed foreign-born nurse providers recruited to American hospitals? What are the roots of the 20th-century American/Philippines nursing relationship? How can an understanding of the historical context of the contemporary relationship between American and Philippines nursing explicate and broaden an understanding of the more general phenomenon of foreign nurse migration?

AMBIGUOUS LEGACY

The relationship between American and Philippine nursing is linked to colonial ties between the two countries and the perception of the Islands' nursing needs prescribed by American physicians, nurses, and others in the health field. Inadequate public health conditions in the Philippines had been reported since the United States' takeover of the islands from Spain in 1898. Contaminated water supplies and poor sewage systems, increased urbanization, insufficient and inefficient basic health care and vaccination programmes, and inept administration were all identified as contributing variables to poor health in the early decades (Heiser, 1909; Lara, 1924; Padua and Tiedeman, 1922).

Nursing and hospital development were established by American missionary workers and medical providers almost immediately after United States possession of the Philippines in an attempt to improve the health conditions of the Filipino people. Most of these early nursing reform efforts were subsidized and sponsored by individual hospitals or by particular interest groups (Giron-Tupas, 1952). As Filipino nurse Anastacia Giron-Tupas wrote in the *History of Nursing in the Philippines* (1952), 'the profession of nursing was unknown before the American occupation' (p. 41).

Early on, the indigenous population was expected to act in partnership with Westernizing efforts. Filipino nurses, sponsored by philanthropic institutions like the Rockefeller Foundation, the Daughters of the American Revolution, and the Catholic Scholarship Fund, for example, were sent to the United States as early as 1911 to further their training and return to the Philippines with American nurse practice views and methods. Anastacia Giron-Tupas, the first Filipino nurse to hold the Philippine General Hospital's chief nurse and superintendent position in the 1920s, for instance, was a 1917 graduate of Philadelphia's Pennsylvania School of Social Work. Her successor, Enriqueta Macaraig, graduated three years later from Teachers College, Columbia University, New York City.

By the 1920s, vigorous worldwide nursing and public health reform were part of the United States' internationalization effort. Rather than sending Filipino nurses to the United States to learn American methods, United States representatives travelled to the Philippines as social and cultural missionaries. The Rockefeller Foundation played a key role in providing funds to internationalize American medical and nursing ideology. Although the Foundation's early nursing reform efforts began with a 'beginning posture of cautious and even skeptical inquiry' (Abrams, 1993, p. 120), the Rockefeller agenda represented one of the first efforts to improve the Islands' overall public health; it serves as an important starting point for an understanding of the contemporary Philippines/American nursing relationship.

As discussed in this article, however, the 1920s Rockefeller campaign to improve public health nursing in the Philippines met with unintended consequences. Rather than improving the public health of the Philippine people or the care rendered to them by nurses, the introduction of American nursing methods and ideas set off a chain of events that may have facilitated the creation of a ready-made workforce for future short-staffed United States hospitals. The later phenomenon of sending for nurses from the Philippines to alleviate American hospital nursing shortages may be partly attributed to the hospitals' central role in health care delivery during this early period of American/Philippines nursing relations. Public health initiatives in the Philippines, not unlike those occurring simultaneously in the United States, transformed into institutional care as economic and social imperatives centred on hospitals and scientific technology (Stevens, 1989).

THE ROCKEFELLER AGENDA

On 7 March 1922 American nurse Alice Fitzgerald set sail on a month-long journey to the Philippine Islands aboard the Army transport ship *Logan*. Commissioned by the International Health Board (IHB) of the Rockefeller Foundation as a 'special member' and nursing adviser on the staff of Philippine Governor-General Leonard Wood, Fitzgerald was charged with, among other things, introducing public health nursing to Philippine Island hospital nursing schools (Minutes of the International Health Board, 1922).

Fitzgerald's two-year assignment, which paid $333.33 per month, was a direct response to American physician Dr Victor Heiser's 1921 Public Health Survey of the Philippines and his exposé of the Islands' alarming prevalence of malaria, tuberculosis, and other contagious diseases as well as escalating infant mortality rates. General Leonard Wood, appointed United States Governor to the Philippines in 1921 by President Warren Harding, commissioned Heiser, the former Director of the Bureau of Health and Chief Quarantine Officer in the Philippines from 1905 to 1914, to study and report the status of public health conditions in the Philippines because Heiser was regarded as 'the expert in Eastern medicine' (Worcester, 1930, p. 2). Heiser's survey, his second complete review of public health conditions in the Islands, included an evaluation of the Philippines health delivery service, the College of Medicine and Surgery, the Bureau of Science, and the facilities for nurse training.

Heiser's recommendations centred on two themes: the persistence of deteriorating standards of health in the Philippines and the necessity for American intervention as a key solution to health care reorganization. Heiser lacked confidence in the Philippine peoples' ability to manage their own affairs. As he put it:

The dead spirit seems to pervade everything. Business men state they can get no action on anything where a Filipino is in charge. I suggest that a person responsible for the nursing service in the Philippines ought to make an inspecting trip to the various places in which nurses are stationed with the hope of stimulating better work.

(Heiser, 1916, p. 570)

Reporting 27,000 annual deaths from malaria and another 50,000 victims of a recent smallpox outbreak, Heiser concluded that 'one of the greatest needs [of the Philippine Health Service] is a more adequate number of properly trained public health nurses' (Heiser, 1921, p. 5). Heiser believed the demand for nursing would increase as the general health of the Filipino people declined and that the few existing schools of nursing were ill-equipped to meet the demand. He argued that an American nurse consultant was necessary to 'give sole attention to the study and improvement of the nursing situation' (Heiser, 1921, p. 6).

Forty-eight-year-old Alice Fitzgerald was an ideal candidate for the nurse consultant position. A 1906 graduate of Johns Hopkins Hospital School of Nursing, Fitzgerald came with considerable experience in international nursing service through the American Red Cross; she had travelled extensively throughout Europe supervising and promoting public health nurse training reform (Noble, 1964). Fitzgerald eagerly accepted the position and the opportunity to introduce Western nursing ideology and practice to the East. As she would remark later in a lecture at Teachers College, Columbia University, New York:

Western ideals in nursing are the guiding star of the East ... the people must be made to see for themselves the advantages to be derived by adopting that which has proven good in the older nursing fields, and when an Easterner has 'seen for himself' and adopts a Western ideal, he rarely wavers from his choice.

(Fitzgerald, 1931, p. 128)

Fitzgerald's view of western superiority would prove to guide most of her perceptions and interventions in Philippine nursing.

AMERICAN NURSING TO THE RESCUE

When Fitzgerald arrived in Manila in April 1922, she immediately laid out her plan to 'visit every hospital and health center and try and meet the people who are doing things in the health line' (Fitzgerald, 1922a). She outlined several major objectives, which together constituted a comprehensive and ambitious agenda for change. Incorporating methods of American professionalism, standardization, and efficiency, Fitzgerald proposed five major reform measures: create a 'central school' for nurses in the Islands; establish a league of nursing education to bring together the directors and instructors of the various nurse training schools in Manila; organize a national nursing association to 'stimulate professional esprit de corps'; study and revise state registration laws and examination methods for nurses; simplify and standard-ize nurse training school methods; and provide medical, nursing, and dental care to rural coasts in the Philippines via a boat mobile health unit (Fitzgerald, 1922b).

Fitzgerald moved quickly and methodically, detailing her first six months' progress in the 'First Report on the Nursing Situation in the Philippine Islands' in 1922. Between April and December 1922, Fitzgerald visited the twelve existing hospital nurse training schools, the Philippine Health Service, and the Public Welfare Commission; established contact with Philippine nursing leaders; helped organize the Philippine Nurses Association; and developed the first public health nursing course at the Philippine General Hospital (PGH), in collaboration with the hospital's chief nurse and superintendent, Miss Anastacia Giron.

Miss Giron was the principal nurse leader in the Philippines and an important liaison between American nursing interests and Philippine nursing reform. International Health Board (IHB) Sec-retary Florence Read encouraged Fitzgerald to forge a relation-ship with Giron, noting, 'it will help matters a great deal if you have her hearty cooperation' (Read, 1922). Fitzgerald reported back to Miss Read that she found Miss Giron 'very cooperative and friendly,' and explained:

I believe we understand each other perfectly as she knows that *I am not here to stay* or to steal any one's job from them. Of course, the fact that I like to work with and for natives does help and I think they readily size up the motives of the workers who come out here.

(Fitzgerald, 1922c)

ORGANIZING CARE THE AMERICAN WAY

Eight of the twelve hospital-based nurse training schools visited by Fitzgerald were located in Manila. The largest, the Philippine General Hospital (PGH), was a 560-bed institution with 260 student and ninety graduate nurses on staff, one-third of whom were male. Its three-year nurse training programme was headed by American-trained Filipino nurses Giron and Enriqueta Macaraig. Fitzgerald was particularly pleased with the hospital's American-influenced general care and nursing leadership, noting, 'PGH stands out conspicuously from every point of view ... [the hospital] could be transferred to any big city in any country and be a credit to it' (Fitzgerald, 1922d, p. 11).

The seven remaining hospital schools in Manila and the four situated in the provinces around the city were considerably smaller than the Philippine General Hospital, were either privately owned or religiously affiliated, and differed from one another in population served, nursing curriculum, and leadership ideologies. Many of the hospital training schools, like PGH, were administered by American-born or American-trained chief nurses. St Luke's Hospital, run by the Episcopal church, for example, employed American chief nurse, Lillian Weiser, and five American and Canadian assistants. The presence of American leadership in conjunction with a Western nursing curriculum confirmed Fitzgerald's confidence that the students would be well trained: 'It is the intention of Dr. Salesby, the hospital director and Miss Weiser to employ American nurses in the capacity of teachers and supervisors ... with this staff of expert teachers and supervisors, the [Filipino] students receive the most thorough and competent training given in Manila' (Fitzgerald, 1922d, p. 6).

Even with an apparent American agenda for nursing and

hospital care, Fitzgerald noted a general lack of communication and training standardization between the different nurse training programmes. Concerned that the future of nursing in the Philippines would be jeopardized by the absence of 'cordial relations' among the various groups, she suggested a mass meeting of all Manila-based institutional nurses. As a result, 200 of the approximately 1,000 graduate nurses in the Philippines met and adopted a plan for a Filipino Nurses Association (FNA). The FNA, modelled after the United States' own League of Nursing Education and American Nurses Association, established three distinct sections for public health nursing, nursing education, and general, private duty and institutional nursing. Philippine nurse Mrs Francesco Delgado was nominated FNA President and American nurses were given 'honorary member' status, although they were able to be active FNA participants (Fitzgerald, 1922e).

FROM ORGANIZATION TO CARE DELIVERY

Fitzgerald (1922d) reported that the worst feature of the health situation in the Philippines was the high infant mortality rate, estimated at 320 deaths per 1,000 live births. She attributed this to a combination of maternal ignorance, poverty, environmental isolation, poor access to health care, shortage of physicians and nurses, and the presence of widespread superstition among the natives, particularly the belief in the evil spirit 'Asuang', deemed 'dangerous' to pregnant women and newborns. Nurses working in public health roles, either through the Philippine Health Service or the Public Welfare Commission, had no formal training and exhibited limited success in child welfare management and the care of patients with yaws, leprosy, and other contagious diseases. Thus Fitzgerald realized that public health nursing education was only one aspect of a complex network of social factors requiring modification. Public health reform, she theorized, was more than simply producing more and better prepared public health nurses. It would involve changing familiar cultural patterns and traditions of health care practice.

Fitzgerald's reform efforts, therefore, largely influenced by her first six months' findings and impressions, attempted to correct nursing deficiencies while casting a wider net around social reform. With this in mind, Fitzgerald accomplished many of her outlined objectives. The first public health nursing course, funded by the Philippine Health Service, began at the Philippine General Hospital on 31 July 1922, with twenty-seven students. Fitzgerald developed the curriculum with the help of Miss Giron and solicited aid in lecturing from many of the physicians she had met while touring hospitals. The curriculum covered an extensive subject matter over a course of six months. Didactic material included 132 hours of public health nursing, 72 hours of preventive medicine and sanitation, 28 hours of vital statistics, 60 hours of charity, 125 hours of home economics, and 72 hours of special lectures.

Almost as soon as the school was operational, however, problems developed. One of the first problems was the school's curriculum. Fitzgerald included mental disease as one of eleven lectures in the special lecture series because she observed substandard care of insane patients in some existing institutions and was convinced that nurses with psychiatric training would be instrumental in improving conditions. She met almost immediate resistance from the Rockefeller Foundation, which deemed the content neither appropriate nor necessary. Historian Raymond B. Fosdick (1952) explained that the Foundation's medical interests were in scientific, measurable, and rational methods of intervention; the non-quantifiable areas of psychiatry and mental disease were not addressed at all by the Foundation until the late 1930s.

Despite the Foundation's obvious resistance, Fitzgerald (1922f) pleaded her case to IHB Secretary, Dr Edwin Embree, in an impassioned letter. Claiming that care of the insane was a responsibility of public health care reform, Fitzgerald wrote:

> You have undoubtedly heard from Dr Heiser and others about the way in which the insane or mentally sick are cared for in the Islands? In the few institutions set aside for this class of patients nothing but custodial care is attempted and it is only since General Wood has been looking into this matter that the chains have been taken off the more violent cases. Until then these poor wretches were chained to the floor until released by death. In the rural villages, I have heard of the mental cases being tied under the nipa hut with the livestock and cared for, if we can use the term, on the same footing with the animals.... If you still feel that this subject should not be included in the curricula at present, I will certainly cut it out of any plans for another course.

IS MORE BETTER?

A second problem involved Fitzgerald's role and relationship with other health officials in the Philippines with whom she often complained of feeling useless and undermined. Commenting to International Health Division General Director, Dr Wickliffe Rose, Fitzgerald (1922g) reported, 'I do not feel that I am of any use whatever to the Governor General for he never refers anything to me either for my opinion or for advice'. Of great concern to Fitzgerald was the question of increasing the numbers of public health nurses. Colonel Munson, Director of the Philippine Health Service, wanted to lower admission standards to nursing schools in response to Governor Wood's 'loud and frequent calls for more and more public health nurses' (Fitzgerald, 1923a).

Munson believed the high school admission standards for nurse training programmes impaired student recruitment, particularly in the non-Christian provinces, and could not see the necessity of placing high educational standards above the needs of the people. Arguing to increase the numbers of nurses rather than the quality of nurses throughout the Islands, Munson wrote to General Wood, 'A Moro girl with a seventh-grade education trained as a nurse would do more good among her own Moro tribe than a much more highly educated Christian girl regarded as an alien by the Moro people' (Munson, 1922).

But increasing the nursing supply, Fitzgerald argued, did not consider the country's financial means to employ them on graduation. Pointing out that 'the increase in the supply of nurses is necessarily dependent upon the economic and financial conditions of the country' Fitzgerald (1923b) argued against efforts to increase nursing numbers at the cost of efficiency. Instead, she advocated ways to secure the necessary funds to create yearly new positions for nurses. 'This gradual increase in demand', she wrote (1923b), 'will be met by a gradual increase in supply.'

In addition to concerns over increasing the supply of nurses too rapidly in a fledgling Philippines economy, Fitzgerald was also unwilling to sacrifice quality for quantity in nursing education. To illustrate her point that lowering admission standards would do nothing for the 'real' problems of nursing distribution and economic instability, Fitzgerald called a meeting with Munson, Philippine Health Service Director Dr Vincente De Jesus, and Dr

Charles Leach. Using survey data from a trip to a province high school in Bagnio, Fitzgerald demonstrated that although provincial girls expressed great interest in nursing, they could not 'be induced to come to the lowlands to study on account of the heat which they dread and because they do not wish to leave their homes' (Fitzgerald, 1922h). Establishing a nurse training school in the mountain provinces, she argued, would attract students, enabling girls to be both well trained, serve local areas in need of nurses, and remain in their own provinces.

Fitzgerald convinced the medical men that short-term solutions might undermine long-range plans for public health improvement and, in fact, successfully developed a nurse training programme in the province of Bagnio in 1923. Furthermore, Fitzgerald induced Governor Wood to send a telegram to all provincial governors encouraging them to hire the sixty-nine new graduates of the second PGH public health nursing course. In his telegram, Wood maintained that the public health nurses, far from being an expense, would be 'wise investments' to the provinces. Despite Fitzgerald's reservations against the rapid increase in the numbers of public health nurses, however, sixty-nine students were admitted to the second public health nursing course in 1923; two-thirds of the graduating nurses were unemployed when a third public health course was considered in July 1923 (Fitzgerald, 1923c).

CONFLICT AND CONSENSUS

Fitzgerald clearly made inroads in some areas, but experienced setbacks in others. Her report of nursing conditions in the Islands failed to capture many of the intrinsic conflicts and tensions that accompanied change implementation. Conflict, in fact, became a regular diet; Fitzgerald's reform efforts were often thwarted or threatened by interpersonal and administrative barriers.

Of major consequence was the falling out between Fitzgerald and her protégé, Anastacia Giron. Against nursing school policy, Giron secretly married Dr Alberto Tupas, an instructor in the College of Medicine and Surgery at the University of Philippines. Once discovered, the newly wedded Mrs Tupas was asked to resign from her position as the PGH Superintendent of Nurses. 'Of course', Fitzgerald asserted in a letter to Dr Heiser, 'a married woman cannot take the position of Superintendent of Nurses as that is certainly a full-time job' (Fitzgerald, 1923d).

The formerly 'friendly and cooperative' Mrs Tupas fuelled Fitz-gerald's anger and mistrust. Writing to Heiser in a letter she 'did not want to dictate to a Filipino', Fitzgerald (1923d) raged, 'I have never before been so disappointed in a person as I thought her a model in all ethical and moral questions and felt she deserved the unique position of leadership which she occupied.' Fitzgerald viewed Giron's marriage as amoral and a threat to her own personal and professional agenda. She opined:

> Miss Giron and her inexcusable behavior came very near wrecking my work as I had spent most of my time strengthening her position and this led her to believe I would continue to back her under 'all circumstances'. . . . I believe Mrs Tupas must be slowly eliminated by pushing Miss [Enriqueta] Maca-raig forward.
>
> (Fitzgerald, 1923e)

Perceiving betrayal, but careful not to attack Tupas openly to give Tupas an 'opportunity of fight' and create a 'split in the ranks', Fitzgerald shifted her loyalties and support to Giron's colleague, Enriqueta Macaraig.

Fitzgerald's views reflected American attitudes that marriage was incompatible with complete devotion to the necessary service and sacrifice of a nursing career. According to biographer Iris Noble (1964), Fitzgerald herself had declined marriage proposals as a young Baltimore debutante in favour of nurse training at Johns Hopkins. But even with her overt anti-marriage sentiments, Fitzgerald made covert concessions because of cultural differences between American and Philippines nurses, especially if nurses were not under the 'protection' of institutional employment. In a confidential addendum to her *Second Annual and Final Report on the Nursing Situation in the PI*, Fitzgerald (1924) noted that 'nurses should not be returned to hospital positions after they are married . . . an exception to this rule can well be made in favor of the public health nurse in the provinces where the protection of a home and husband is an advantage' (p. 19).

By December 1923, most of the PGH's second class of public health nurses secured employment. But rising anti-male senti-ments by the American-run Red Cross and Public Welfare Com-mission threatened the employment of the nearly one-third male graduates. Although generally unsupportive of male nurses, Fitz-gerald made a second concession based on cultural difference, viewing men as valuable adjuncts to public health nursing in the Philippines. 'Though I do not believe male nurses are necessary in other countries', Fitzgerald (1923e) commented to Heiser, 'I do feel that for the present at least there are many isolated districts where it would not be right to send a young woman and where the male nurses can do good work'. Male Filipino nurses, like married nurses in remote districts, were exceptions to West-ern-based rules of appropriate nurse gender and marital status; concerns with safety in the uncivilized terrain of the Philippine Islands took precedence over convention.

HISTORICAL ROOTS AND CONTEMPORARY LINKAGES

Although the United States' formal decolonization and severance of political ties with the Philippine Islands occurred almost five decades ago (1946), the social, cultural, political, and economic links between the former colony and its mother country were clearly not surrendered. American influence and intervention in Philippines nursing affairs spanned the century; preparation of nurses by Western standards created an oversupply of nurses with hospital and technological expertise who were ill-prepared to respond to the Islands' public health needs. Moreover, appropri-ate funding was never earmarked for public health nursing services such that nurses prepared for public health roles often had difficulty securing positions.

With an excess in nurse production and limited economic capa-bility for postgraduate hiring in the 1950s, Filipino nurses faced widespread unemployment. Attracted by invitations to participate in study, observation, and/or employment opportunities in the United States and other industrialized nations experiencing post-war nursing shortages, Filipino nurses began to look abroad for professional opportunities. Between 1956 and 1973, for example, 12,526 Filipino nurses entered the United States through the Exchange Visitor Program (Alinea and Senador, 1973). Later, nurses were directly recruited by agencies and hospitals for pri-marily hospital-based employment. After 1965, the numbers of emigrating nurses grew dramatically. New American immigration policies lifted previous restrictions on Asian immigration; Filipino nurses practising in United States hospitals increased by 400 per cent between 1965 and 1972 alone (Mejia et al., 1979).

In response to the demand for Filipino nurse labour in American hospitals, numbers of nursing schools in the Philippines rose from 17 in 1950, to 46 in 1965, to 88 in 1974 (Ortin, 1990). Numbers of registered Filipino nurses increased exponentially from 7,000 in 1948 to over 57,000 25 years later (Sotejo, 1974). This trend led once more to widespread nurse unemployment in the 1970s, exacerbated by the Philippines' declining economic state under Ferdinand Marcos. Subjected to ambivalent and dichotomous messages, nurses were simultaneously encouraged to emigrate and remit wages home to strengthen the national economy and chastised for leaving home and placing their personal and family's economic interests above nationalism (Marcos, 1974; Castillejos, 1966; Castrence, 1966). Nevertheless, nurses continued to immigrate to United States hospitals to seek occupational and educational opportunities.

Nurses in the Philippines continue to be educated according to Western nursing standards that emphasize hospital-based care over community-based practice despite decaying public health conditions in the Philippines. As the anonymous author of an article called 'FNG Exodus, Why?' put it in 1986, 'nurse training gears nurses to the Western thrust of care rather than the prevention of disease' (p. 2). Infant mortality rates today hover at 52.9 deaths per 1,000 live births and high morbidity and mortality from tuberculosis, diarrhoea, and nutritional deficiencies top the nation's health problems.

There is still concern that the production of nurses outweighs the needs and the economy of the country. Cries of 'brain drain' ring familiar as nurses are siphoned to industrial nations, particularly the United States. American hospitals represent the continuation of the colonial relationship by its overwhelming hegemony in the health care systems of both the former colony and its colonizer. Of course, many other factors play important roles in nurses' decisions to migrate abroad – better pay and working conditions and the ability to remit earnings home have been repeatedly cited.

SUMMARY

The Rockefeller's early public health initiatives in the Philippine Islands created an unintended impetus for the continuing preparation of large numbers of Filipino nurse caregivers for hospitals in industrial nations. West Germany, the United States, Canada, and, more recently, Saudi Arabia have all benefited from the ongoing production and exportation of Western-trained nurses from the Philippines.

Fitzgerald was one of a number of exogenous reformers invited or commissioned by various groups to change existing indigenous cultural and social systems throughout the world. Preaching a gospel of models, principles, and techniques derived from American nursing experience that she believed would uplift and profit Filipino nurses and the Philippines' public health, Fitzgerald was driven by an unflagging faith in the virtue of her commitment to export America's superior values and doctrines to an uncivilized people. Thus, although sympathetic to the Filipino people and acutely aware of the cultural differences between the two countries, Fitzgerald, like other reform-minded women, subscribed to the notion of superiority of her own cultural and political system. Viewing nursing as rational, scientific, and universalistic, Fitzgerald defined appropriate public health nursing intervention in opposition to the presumed irrationality and superstitions of Filipino customs and beliefs that were essentially obstacles to be overcome.

Health care reform was one avenue for infusing American ideals into the 'less privileged' colony. The Rockefeller agenda provided the means for extending this 'benevolent assimilation', a term coined by President McKinley guaranteeing the Filipino people 'happiness, peace, and prosperity' in exchange for their submission to American values and virtues (Karnow, 1989, p. 14). Under the veneer of moral rectitude, efforts to reform health care sought to Americanize Filipino nursing and health delivery rather than Filipinize American nurses and other health workers in the Philippines.

Nursing is not alone in this respect. Parallel arguments and observations have been applied in other disciplines. John Bryant's (1965) report to the Rockefeller Foundation on the education of physicians in developing countries is a good example. Much as Fitzgerald viewed Western nursing as the stimulus to good nursing care throughout the world, Bryant noted:

Modern medicine is a product of the Western part of the world. It evolved in the West to fit the needs of the West . . . . Relatively little has been changed by the trans-oceanic passage.

The medical schools in the developing world have Western curricula and Western ideas of excellence. The apparent goal is to produce a doctor who is good in the same sense that the West tries to define good.

The Philippine public health nursing story and subsequent nurse emigration to American hospitals represents the historical legacy of colonialism and how implanted institutions come to function more in accordance with the needs of imperialist powers over colonized nations. More broadly, the rapid production of nurses in the Philippines for exportation to the United States reflects the wider problem faced by many lesser industrialized nations whose limited resources make them ill-equipped to prepare adequate numbers and types of health care providers to care for the health care problems of their indigenous populations.

NOTE

1 This chapter is republished with kind permission of Sage Publications and the *Western Journal of Nursing Research*, 1995, 17 (5) pp. 540–55.

REFERENCES

Abrams, S.E. (1993) Brilliance and bureaucracy: Nursing and changes in the Rockefeller Foundation, 1915–1930, *Nursing History Review*, 1, 119–137.

Alinea, P.G. and Senador, G.B. (1973) Leaving for abroad ... here's a word of caution, *Philippine Journal of Nursing*, 17, 141–147.

American Nurses' Association (1951) Study programmes and employment arranged for foreign nurses who are at present in the U.S.A., American Nurses' Association Collection, No. N87, Box 180, Nursing Archives, Boston University, Mugar Library, Boston, MA.

Brush, B.L. (1993) Exchangees or employees? The exchange visitor program and foreign nurse immigration to the United States, 1945–1990, *Nursing History Review*, 1, 171–180.

Brush, B.L. (1994) Sending for nurses: Foreign nurse immigration to American hospitals, 1945–1980, unpublished doctoral dissertation, University of Pennsylvania, Philadelphia.

Bryant, J. (1965) The education of physicians in developing countries. Margaret G. Arnstein Collection, Box 8, Folder 69, Boston University, Mugar Library, Boston, MA.

Castillejos, E.B. (1966) The exchange visitor program: Report and recommendation, *Philippine Journal of Nursing*, 35, 306–307.

Castrence, P.S. (1966) Challenge to the Filipino nurses, *Philippine Journal of Nursing*, 35, 205–207.

Fitzgerald, A. (1922a) Letter to Florence Read, 23 April. R.G. 1.1, 242 C, Box 5, Folder 47, Rockefeller Archive Center, North Tarrytown, New York.

Fitzgerald, A. (1922b) Letter to Victor Heiser, 22 May. R.G. 1.1, 242 C, Box 5, Folder 47, Rockefeller Archive Center, North Tarrytown, New York.

Fitzgerald, A. (1922c) Letter to Florence Read, 25 June. R.G. 1.1, 242 C, Box 5, Folder 47, Rockefeller Archive Center, North Tarrytown, New York.

Fitzgerald, A. (1922d) Report on the nursing situation in the Philippine Islands, April to December, 1922. R.G. 1.1, 242 C, Box 5, Folder 52, Rockefeller Archive Center, North Tarrytown, New York.

Fitzgerald, A. (1922e) Letter to Wickliffe Rose, 9 September. R.G. 1.1, 242 C, Box 5, Folder 48, Rockefeller Archive Center, North Tarrytown, New York.

Fitzgerald, A. (1922f) Letter to Edwin Embree, 10 August. R.G. 1.1. 242 C, Box 5, Folder 48, Rockefeller Archive Center, North Tarrytown, New York.

Fitzgerald, A. (1922g) Letter to Wickliffe Rose, 19 November. R.G. 1.1, 242 C, Box 5, Folder 48, Rockefeller Archive Center, North Tarrytown, New York.

Fitzgerald, A. (1922h) Letter to Vincente De Jesus, 4 December. Box 5, Folder 52, Rockefeller Archive Center, North Tarrytown, New York.

Fitzgerald, A. (1923a) Letter to Victor Heiser, 7 June. R.G. 1.1, 242 C, Box 5, Folder 48, Rockefeller Archive Center, North Tarrytown, New York.

Fitzgerald, A. (1923b) Memorandum concerning the supply of nurses in the Philippine Islands. R.G. 1.1, 242 C, Box 5, Folder 49, Rockefeller Archive Center, North Tarrytown, New York.

Fitzgerald, A. (1923c) Letter to Victor Heiser, 3 September. R.G. 1.1., 242 C, Box 5, Folder 49, Rockefeller Archive Center, North Tarrytown, New York.

Fitzgerald, A. (1923d) Letter to Victor Heiser, 9 November. R.G. 1.1., 242 C, Box 5, Folder 49, Rockefeller Archive Center, North Tarrytown, New York.

Fitzgerald, A. (1923e) Letter to Victor Heiser, 28 December. R.G. 1.1., 242 C, Box 5, Folder 49, Rockefeller Archive Center, North Tarrytown, New York.

Fitzgerald, A. (1924) *Second Annual and Final Report on the Nursing Situation in the Philippine Islands – January 1, 1923–January 1*, 1924. R.G. 1.1., Box 5, Folder 54, Rockefeller Archive Center, North Tarrytown, New York.

Fitzgerald, A. (1931, February/April) Western influences on nursing education in the orient. Paper presented at the meeting of the International Aspects of Nursing Education, Teachers' College, Columbia University, New York, NY.

FNG exodus: Why? (1986) *UGAT: Newsletter of the Philippine Center for Immigrant Rights*, 1, 2.

Fosdick, R.B. (1952) *The Story of the Rockefeller Foundation*, New York: Harper & Brothers.

Giron-Tupas, A. (1952) *History of Nursing in the Philippines*, Manila, Philippines: Author.

Gonzales, N.A. (1989) Let us nurse our society back to health., *Philippine Journal of Nursing*, 59, 11–14.

Heiser, V.G. (1909) Sanitation in the Philippine Islands since American occupations, with particular reference to reduction in mortality by elimination of intestinal parasites, especially uncinaria, *Journal of the American Medical Association*, 52, 97–99.

Heiser, V.G. (1916) Notes of 1916 trip, Vol. II. R.G. 5, Series 2, International Health Board, Rockefeller Archive Center, North Tarrytown, New York.

Heiser, V.G. (1921) Suggested program for improving present health conditions. R.G. 5, Series 242 C, Box 20, Folder 127, Rockefeller Archive Center, North Tarrytown, New York.

Karnow, S. (1989) *In Our Image: America's Empire in the Philippines*, New York: Ballantine.

Lara, H. (1924) The cause of the unusually high rate of prevalence of typhoid fever in the city of Manila. R.G. 1.1., 242 C, Box 20, Folder 123, Rockefeller Archive Center, North Tarrytown, New York.

Marcos, Ferdinand E. (1974) Address, *Philippine Journal of Nursing*, 43, 13–23.

Mejia, A., Pizurki, H. and Royston, E. (1979) *Physician and Nurse Migration: Analysis and Policy Implications*, Geneva: World Health Organization.

Minutes of the International Health Board (1922) Appointment of Miss Alice Fitzgerald. R.G. 1.1, 242 C, Box 5, Folder 47, Rockefeller Archive Center, North Tarrytown, New York.

Munson, E.L. (1922) Letter to Leonard Wood, 7 October. R.G. 5, 242 C, Box 20, Folder 126, Rockefeller Archive Center, North Tarrytown, New York.

Noble, I. (1964) *Nurse Around the World: Alice Fitzgerald*, New York: Julian Messner.

Ortin, E.L. (1990) The brain drain as viewed by an exporting country, *International Nursing Review*, 37, 340–344.

Padua, R.G. and Tiedeman, W.D. (1922) Preliminary report on the malaria situation in the province of Laguna. R.G. 1.1., Series 242, Box 20, Folder 124, Rockefeller Archive Center, North Tarrytown, New York.

Read, F. (1922) Letter to Alice Fitzgerald, 20 May. R.G. 1.1, 242C, Box 5, Folder 47, Rockefeller Archive Center, North Tarrytown, New York.

Sotejo, J.V. (1974) Time to integrate, *Philippine Journal of Nursing*, 43, 183, 221.

Stevens, R. (1989) *In Sickness and in Wealth: American Hospitals in the Twentieth Century*, New York: Basic Books.

United States General Accounting Office (1989) *Information on Foreign Nurses Working in the United States under Temporary Work Visas*, Washington, DC: U.S. Government Printing Office.

Worcester, D.C. (1930) *The Philippines Past and Present*, New York: Macmillan.

Chapter 4

Rescue and redemption
The rise of female medical missions in colonial India during the late nineteenth and early twentieth centuries

Rosemary Fitzgerald

INTRODUCTION

At the turn of the twentieth century, the subject of medical missions conjured up, for a large British audience, the image of heroic doctors and nurses applying the balm of western medicine to suffering humanity in god-forsaken corners of the globe. The medical missionary, especially the *lady* medical missionary, was an icon of the mission movement, appealing even to sceptical Christians, who could identify with the humanitarianism if not the evangelism of the medical mission project. Writing in 1897, the Reverend Geoffrey Lefroy of the Cambridge Mission to Delhi observed:

> probably there is no branch of Mission Work which appeals more widely to popular sympathies or receives more ready and ungrudging help than that which addresses itself to the relief of sickness ... in lands where western science, western methods, and western tenderness and care have not yet pene-trated.[1]

The mission contribution to the display of western medical ideas, institutions and practices, and the part that women mission-aries played in this display, gained particular significance in the context of colonial India. Under colonial health policies the pro-vision of medical relief to the mass of the Indian population was woefully inadequate, and most conspicuously so in the case of Indian women.[2] Western responses to Indian women's health needs came largely from philanthropic organizations and, most notably, the missionary societies. While the colonial adminis-tration's commitment to the issue of Indian women's health was slow to emerge and never more than limited, missions developed energetic and often innovative approaches to this subject. Even as late as 1927, when government health services for women had begun to be developed more widely, the ninety-three mission hospitals for women represented over half of all women's hospitals in India; missions were also providing 102 schools for the training of nurses while only fifty-five government nursing schools had been established.[3]

This chapter explores the rise of female medical missions – mission medicine carried out exclusively for and by women – in colonial India and the development of this work by Protestant missionary societies in the later nineteenth and early twentieth centuries. During this period women's medical mission work became a highly prominent arena of missionary activity in India, providing a sharp contrast with the first half of the nineteenth century when neither medicine nor women missionaries had occupied an official place in the mission crusade.

THE RISE OF MEDICINE IN THE ARSENAL OF MISSIONARY METHODS

At the birth of the modern foreign mission movement in the 1790s and early 1800s, medical concerns occupied only a marginal place in the mission agenda. For the following half century or more, missionary societies continued to register scant interest in establishing medical work as an arm of missionary service overseas. The Edinburgh Medical Missionary Society, one of the earliest organizations to expound the value of medicine as a missionary strategy, reported that before 1841, the year of the Society's foundation, only three British missionaries were officially engaged in medical work overseas. At the close of 1852, the Edinburgh Society's Annual Report estimated that there were no more than thirteen European medical missionaries employed by the various Protestant missionary societies.[4]

In these early years of mission organization, the mainline missionary societies expressed a clear preference for the appointment of ordained men as missionaries. The missionary's paramount commission was to 'elevate the mind and save the soul' through the direct evangelism of preaching and teaching. The few medical men engaged by mission boards were primarily recruited in an attempt to safeguard the health of missionaries and their families in mission fields where the attrition rate, through death and disease, was felt to be unacceptably high. If medical candidates for mission service remained unordained, they were not, strictly speaking, thought of as missionaries; they were more likely to be regarded as the clerical missionary's lay assistant.[5]

A reappraisal of the role of medicine in the mission enterprise, and recognition of the special place and power of medical missionaries in the mission campaign, came about gradually, and not without struggle, only in the later decades of the nineteenth century. A number of parallel developments prompted the shift of medical work from the fringes to the centre of mission attention during this period.

First, there was growing awareness that medical work might act as an 'entering wedge' that offered tactical advantages in fields overtly hostile to mission penetration.[6] Mission stations reported that initial attempts to carry out medical work had proved 'a most powerful weapon in breaking down prejudice and animosity' and 'a means of opening doors which would otherwise have remained shut'.[7]

Second, efforts to create a space for medical work in the repertoire of missionary methods were supported by the social and scientific changes occurring in medical education and practice during the second half of the nineteenth century. The professional consolidation of medicine, together with advances in medical science and improvements in diagnosis and therapeutics, created a more favourable climate for those pressing for the inclusion of medical work within the mission agenda.

Finally, a more substantial and less grudging legitimation was granted to medical work in the mission context by the changing mission theology of the later nineteenth century. The earlier 'muscular Christianity' of direct evangelism began to give way to an expanded theology of mission that included indirect as well as direct forms of evangelism. The mission task came to be seen as centring on the social as well as the spiritual, on the concerns of this life as well as the next. Medical missions appeared supremely well-suited to this new definition of the mission project in terms of the opportunities they claimed to offer for achieving 'the double cure' – the relief of physical suffering *and* the saving of the 'sin-sick soul'.[8]

By the early twentieth century medical mission work had come to be seen as of strategic importance in 'the delivery of a "frontal attack" upon the forces of error and superstition', particularly in those 'hard and stubborn' fields, such as India and China, where years of 'patient endeavour and dreary waiting' had produced few tangible results.[9] During the 1840s and 1850s only a handful of Protestant medical missionaries were at work worldwide; by the end of the century the number of medically-qualified Protestant missionaries had risen to 680.[10] In 1899, Protestant missions around the world were reported to be running 379 hospitals, 783 dispensaries, and over sixty medical and nursing schools.[11]

India, together with China, dominated the medical mission landscape. Only seven medical missionaries were posted in India in 1858, but this figure climbed to twenty-eight in 1882, 140 in 1895, and 280 in 1905.[12] By 1916, when the Protestant medical mission force worldwide had grown to 1,052 doctors and 537 nurses, 281 (27 per cent) of the missionary doctors were serving in India, 420 (40 per cent) in China. These two mission fields accounted for 44 per cent of all missionary nurses – 108 (20 per cent) were to be found in India, 127 (24 per cent) in China.[13] No other mission fields attracted such high proportions of the medical mission force.

By 1916, missions in India were running 183 hospitals and 376 dispensaries that provided treatment for over one-and-a-quarter million patients annually.[14] Women played a vital role in the development of this avenue of mission work in India, although an officially acknowledged place for women in the male bastions of missions, medicine and empire was neither readily granted nor easily achieved.

'THE NOBLE MISSION OF WOMEN TO WOMEN'

Before the 1860s, the main mission societies were extremely reluctant to appoint women as missionaries. However, long before women were officially admitted to the missionary ranks, they had accompanied male missionaries overseas as their female kin.[15] Mission boards generally accepted, indeed even encouraged, women's presence in the mission field, provided they were there by virtue of their domestic responsibilities towards male missionaries.

Apart from the comforts that women were seen to bring to the home lives of male missionaries, women also served a more public function for the mission project by demonstrating to indigenous audiences the domestic arrangements and gender relations of the western Christian family. However, in taking a place within the mission station as the 'incorporated' female relatives of male missionaries, women were more than simply passive exemplars of the Christian domestic model.[16] From their earliest days in the mission field, women had ventured beyond the boundaries of their own domestic space to publicize Christian domestic culture in a more active sense. They did so by engaging in basic educational and medical work among local women and children, often carried out from the verandah of the mission bungalow or, by home visitation, within the households of indigenous society. The domestic character of this work, together with its focus on indigenous women and children, ensured that the gendering of mission activity maintained a formal adherence to the separation of spheres. Men occupied the salaried position of the official missionary engaged in public evangelism; women undertook the unpaid ancillary work of domestic evangelism. Women's activities in the mission field could be read as 'truly womanly work, not taking us out of our sphere as mothers, and wives, and sisters, but binding us even more closely to the home consecration [sic], that those in heathen lands may have the blessings that we have'.[17] Women of the mission family were authorized – by their 'natural' identification with domesticity and maternalism, by their Christian credentials and by the assumed authority of their race – to carry the qualities of 'True Christian Womanhood' into the households of the heathen world through the medium of what came to be known as 'women's work for women'.[18]

As the nineteenth century progressed, mission bodies increasingly came to recognize that 'women's work' might prove to be of central rather than incidental value to the mission project. 'Women's work for women' was progressively elevated from the province of the missionary's female relatives to a subject of special mission interest that demanded the deployment of single women as fully accredited missionaries. This move was prompted by several developments that gathered momentum over the second half of the century. First, this period witnessed the rise of women's missionary societies and auxiliaries and a larger voice for women in mission polity at the 'home base' in the west; second, the disappointing results reported from some of the most significant and long-standing mission fields suggested the need to consider new methods of work, such as the use of female agents;

and third, women were assumed to possess an 'instinctive' capacity for compassion and caring and a 'natural' aptitude for philanthropic work, qualities that matched the emphasis on humanitarianism in the new theology of missions.

The example of the first women's missionary organizations, and their reports of 'women's work for women' from the field, gradually persuaded the main mission boards that female agency might offer new and irresistible opportunities for mission work, especially among 'the secluded women of the East'. The boards also recognized that 'the women's part of the work' could not be expanded solely on the basis of the informal labour of missionary wives, sisters and daughters. The formal development of 'women's work for women' necessitated the adoption of unmarried women into the official missionary ranks as fully accredited 'career' missionaries.

From the 1860s onwards an increasing number of women joined the missionary force; by 1888, over 1,000 European and American women were reported to be serving as missionaries overseas.[19] By 1910, the Protestant churches worldwide reported that the total mission force of over 19,000 comprised 4,988 unmarried women (excluding physicians), 5,406 missionary wives (excluding physicians), 341 women physicians (marital status unspecified) and 8,545 men.[20] Although women missionaries were to be found in many 'faraway outposts of the world', they were most heavily concentrated in the mission fields of India and China. In 1910, 28 per cent of unmarried, non-medical women missionaries were posted in India; 22 per cent in China.[21] No other fields attracted such high proportions of the female mission force. Medical women entering missionary service were most likely to be destined for India or China – of the 341 women missionary doctors serving in 1910, half were to be found in India and one-third in China.

WOMEN'S WORK FOR WOMEN IN INDIA – THE CENTRALITY OF THE ZENANA

The most compelling evidence for the need to develop women's mission work had come from those areas of the non-Christian world where strong traditions of female seclusion presented insuperable barriers to male missionary methods. In India it was apparent that the evangelism of male missionaries would never reach those women whose lives were framed by the conventions of purdah. Strictly secluded women were prohibited from entering the public arena – the theatre of male missionary methods – while the zenana, the exclusively female quarters within the Indian household, remained beyond the bounds of male missionary intrusion. However, the work of the early mission women suggested that female agents could reach into this previously uncolonized domestic space and reveal to the mission gaze what lay hidden in its recesses – 'the inner social life of India'.[22]

Access to the zenana, this inner region of the Indian household, became a central focus of mission attention; female mission agents and their 'women's work for women' promised to offer a key to the door of the 'hearts and homes' of India. This avenue of mission work was made particularly significant by social and regional variations in the practice of women's seclusion in India. Seclusion practices were observed most strongly by the upper echelons of the Hindu community and by broad sections of the Muslim population; women's seclusion was also more evident in the north, north-western and eastern parts of the country.[23] These were the social and geographic regions where male missionary efforts to gather converts had proved least successful. 'Women's work for women' appeared to offer a novel and more penetrating route into these unreached areas that had remained resistant to male missionary approach. Above all, work by women for women appeared to present a unique opportunity to enter the influential 'better classes' of Indian society where missions expected the introduction of Christianity to act as a catalyst that would produce far-reaching social as well as personal transformation.

The 'storming of the zenana' began in the 1850s and gathered strength as growing numbers of women missionaries were sent out, 'with their weapons of love, tact and sympathy', to broaden the assault.[24] As the titles of many of the early women's missionary organizations suggest, the first formal overtures towards the zenana were made primarily through the means of educational work. However, the first wave of female missionaries frequently had to report that, especially in the households of the higher classes, zenana doors remained 'fast shut'.

Addressing British mission circles in the early 1870s, Dr William Elmslie, a noted medical missionary in Kashmir, pointed out that 'millions of the women of the middle and upper classes of India are unapproachable through the agency of education'.[25] Elmslie wrote:

> Is there no other key but that of education with which to open the door to the inner social life of India? We think there is certainly one other such key and that key is female medical missions ... the practice of medicine by a lady, for the purpose of not merely curing, but of Christianizing her patients. ... This is the key which may be said to fit every lock ... there are few, if any, homes into which the lady medical missionary would not be heartily welcomed. ... She would find an entrance where the educational missionary would find the door closed.[26]

The prohibitions of purdah largely excluded male medical practitioners from treating secluded women; medical access to the zenana could only be achieved through female agents who, in the mission view, were given 'the special honour ... to enter the domestic Bastilles of the East with healing and light, and to make an end ... of the barbarous practices of native midwifery, and of the many remediable sufferings of their own sex'.[27] Western Christian women were urged to 'giv[e] up home and [go] to India, to nurse and doctor their needy and suffering sisters, *for Christ's sake*'.[28]

Within mission discourse, the cause of female medical missions was advanced through the representation of the zenana as a domain offering exceptional opportunities for the demonstration of 'the double cure' – the healing of body and soul. Zenana women were seen as in the most acute need of both 'rescue and redemption' for they were regarded by the missions, paradoxically, not only as powerless victims of medical neglect and maltreatment but also as powerful guardians of indigenous culture and religious tradition. Secluded woman were depicted as pitiful prisoners, 'cabined, cribbed, [and] confined' within zenana walls.[29] However, they were also seen as the 'zealous adherent[s] of traditional heathenism' and, as wives, mothers, and grandmothers, 'mighty counter-influences' capable of erasing the effects of missionary work among Indian men.[30] In gaining access to women within the 'darkened recesses of the heathen home', it was held that:

> Medical Missions by women and for women are destined to

do far more than bring the balm of healing to many a poor sufferer. They are calculated to exert an influence which goes to the very springs of the life of the nation purifying it at its source and centre.[31]

The high proportion of women missionary doctors and nurses sent to India reflects the significance of their work for the mission project there. At the turn of the twentieth century, there were 711 missionary doctors (489 male, 222 female) serving in Protestant missions worldwide.[32] From this medical force, 169 were posted to India, 81 men and 88 women.[33] By 1916, the worldwide Protestant medical mission force stood at 1,052 doctors (743 male, 309 female), and 537 nurses; 159 (51 per cent) of the women doctors and 108 (20 per cent) of the nurses were deployed in India.[34] China was the only other mission field that came close to rivalling India's attraction for women missionary doctors and nurses.[35]

FROM 'PILLBOX' TO PROFESSIONAL PRACTICE – THE DEVELOPMENT OF FEMALE MEDICAL MISSION WORK

Initially, female medical mission work relied on women who possessed little more than 'medicine chests, commonsense and the wisdom that experience soon began to give'.[36] However, by the closing decades of the nineteenth century, the claim that medicine had to its own distinct place and power in the mission field demanded that medical mission work distance itself from these earlier 'pillbox' practices.

Growing confidence in medical and nursing innovations accomplished in the West inspired the search for a more assured and prestigious place for medical work in the mission project, and the conviction that this realm of missionary labour should reflect professional forms of western practice. The development of mission medicine in the later nineteenth century was marked by a shift away from the unregulated, informal 'pillbox' medicine of earlier years, towards more systematic, formalized modes of work. This change was reflected in the demise of the 'amateur' physicians and nurses of former days and increasing insistence that medical mission work belonged, not to the general missionary, but to the professionally qualified missionary doctor and, eventually, nurse.

In India and elsewhere, the transformation of female medical missions was a gradual but inexorable process. When the first female medical missions were initiated, in the 1860s and 1870s, their progress was hampered by the uncertain character of the nursing and medical skills available in the missions. At a time when nursing reform was in its infancy, the description in mission records of women applicants possessing a 'nursing background' covered a multitude of different levels of knowledge, skill and experience.

Given the pre-eminence of the professionally qualified physician in the new era of mission medicine, women's lack of access to medical education presented an even thornier problem. The early advocates of female medical missions rejected, in the strongest terms, any suggestion that women should join male students in the existing medical courses and recommended that 'until there is a medical school for ladies, the necessary professional instruction ought to be given to the lady missionary in a private manner'.[37] Such recommendations were open to diverse interpretation and many improvised methods were resorted to in the attempt to equip women missionaries for medical work overseas. There were, however, growing fears that, in carrying out medical and even surgical procedures, 'half-educated lady-doctors' and 'partially trained' women were smudging the boundaries between nursing and medical work and in danger of bringing female medical missions into disrepute by remaining perilously close to the unregulated and inferior practices of the 'pillbox' medicine of the past.

The opening of medical education to women in the West finally gave women missionaries the opportunity to obtain the complete medical training that was increasingly seen as crucial for the full efficiency and effectiveness of medical work in the mission field. In Britain, the founding of the London School of Medicine for Women in 1874, and of three more women's medical schools in 1886, 1888 and 1890, provided single-sex institutions that enabled women missionaries to become medically qualified under conditions acceptable to mission sensibilities. Fanny Butler, one of the first students to enrol at the London School, entered the Medical Register in Britain in 1880, and immediately set sail for India, under the auspices of the Church of England Zenana Missionary Society, as the first medically qualified British woman missionary. She was not, however, the first medically qualified woman missionary to reach India. That distinction belonged to an American – Dr Clara Swain had arrived in 1869, as the first fully accredited woman physician sent out by any missionary society to the non-Christian world.

The arrival of medical women carrying the authority of professional qualifications laid the basis for a more elaborate division of labour between nursing and medical work within female medical missions. Women missionaries with full medical qualifications were able to claim the title of 'medical missionary' – a designation that was increasingly restricted to those who 'have systematically studied medicine and surgery, and have obtained legal qualifications to practise'.[38] The woman medical missionary was seen as occupying a 'more inviting and influential sphere of usefulness' than her less privileged colleague – the missionary nurse.[39] John Lowe's influential treatise on medical missions was explicit in stating:

> There cannot be too many thoroughly well-trained nurses sent out to work amongst the women and children in our mission fields ... but ... do not designate as *medical missionaries* such partially trained agents, and thus lead the inmates of the Zenanas to expect from them services which they are not qualified to render.[40]

Missionary nurses were regarded as 'invaluable assistants' who should 'lay claim to no higher functions' and be content to go about their 'unpretentious but useful work' in 'a quiet, unostentatious way'.[41]

Although nurses were initially overshadowed by the entrance of women doctors into medical mission work, the opening years of the twentieth century saw the development of a much more positive evaluation of the missionary nurse and her sphere. The nurse was no longer categorized as 'partially trained' – as measured by the yardstick of medical qualifications. She was judged by the quality of her nursing training and the measure of her nursing qualifications. In the British *Missionary Directory for Nurses*, published in 1908, the mission societies' requirements for missionary nurse candidates indicated an almost universal demand for a full three-year course of training in a recognized school, plus the desirability of additional qualifications in areas such as midwifery, dispensing and tropical diseases.[42] The time had passed when nursing work was seen as an intuitive feminine accomplishment that any woman in the mission field might care to exercise. The call was now for the restriction of the title 'missionary nurse' to those with 'the very best and fullest professional qualifications' who would not falter in their demonstration of the superior nursing skills of the West. The designation no longer belonged to 'missionary ladies who have obtained a smattering of nursing or have become qualified in just one branch of the nursing profession'.[43]

Although the woman doctor still took precedence in the hierarchy of the female medical mission, the rising numbers of fully trained missionary nurses arriving in India in the first decade of this century could feel confident that there was a widely expressed need for the trained nurse and an increasing appreciation of her services.[44] In 1910 Dr Jenny Muller, of St Stephen's Mission Hospital in Delhi, reported: 'It is no exaggeration to say that in India today the call for nurses is much louder than that for women doctors.'[45] Nurses were urgently needed to staff the hospitals for women and children that were rapidly replacing the attendance of female patients in their own homes. As Dr Muller exclaimed: 'We cannot have Hospitals without nurses – in the present day!'[46] The appeal for nurses with the 'best' and 'widest' qualifications reflected the mission view that missionary nurses were destined not only to undertake difficult and demanding nursing work but also to serve as educators of a new generation of Indian nurses. Paramount importance was attached to the need for missionary nurses to develop the training of Indian women and to lay the basis of an Indian nursing profession modelled on the styles and standards of nursing in the West.

The missions were aware that they could 'never by themselves alone touch more than a fringe of suffering womanhood' in fields as vast as India.[47] The scale of the task to 'rescue and redeem' India's women demanded that the missionaries turn their attention to the medical and nursing training of local women to supplement the medical mission force and ensure the continuation and expansion of the work. Missionaries were also conscious that training Indian women as doctors and as nurses offered opportunities to exert Christian influence over women's medical and nursing education in India. Missions anticipated that this work would eventually be taken up by 'native governments' and that, if no strong foundations inspired by Christianity had been laid, it would then be instituted 'under conditions unfavourable to the highest moral and religious ideals'.[48] By the early twentieth century, missionary medicine viewed one of its primary responsibilities as the teaching and training of indigenous doctors and nurses in a Christian atmosphere that would imbue their future professional practice with an ethos of selfless service and devotion to duty rather than with a spirit of 'commercialism'.[49]

CONCLUSION

During the later decades of the nineteenth century missionary medicine moved from the periphery of mission activity to become one of the central strategies of the mission enterprise. In this same period female missionaries were acknowledged as playing a vital role in bringing missions into contact with the women of other lands. When that contact was established through medical and nursing care delivered by western women to their 'less fortunate sisters overseas', it was believed to provide one of the most effective methods of reaching and touching the lives of women, especially secluded women, in the non-Christian world. By the early twentieth century western women's medical and nursing work in the mission field was celebrated as one of the most valuable spheres of missionary endeavour.

As the twentieth century progressed, the preparation and training of local people who would become medical missionaries in their own lands became 'one of the cardinal elements in the entire medical missionary plan of campaign'.[50] Women missionary doctors and nurses were among those spearheading the efforts to establish and develop formal programmes for training Indian women in western medical and nursing practice. Although the mission contribution to Indian women's medical education was far from negligible, women's medical mission work within India became most closely associated with the development of nursing education. The growth of the nursing profession in India during the early half of this century lies beyond the scope of this chapter but an indication of the part played by missions in the history of Indian nursing is illustrated by the fact that, at the time of World War II, some 90 per cent of Indian nurses came from the small Christian community, and 80 per cent of all Indian nurses had been trained in mission hospitals.[51] The prominent influence of the missions in shaping the Indian nursing field continued up to and beyond India's independence and proved to be one of the most enduring legacies of the female medical missions of the colonial era.

NOTES

1 G.A. Lefroy, 'A Plea for Medical Missions', *Short Papers of the Society for the Propagation of the Gospel and the Cambridge Mission to Delhi*, No. 2, 1897, p. 1, Cambridge Brotherhood Library, Delhi.
2 See, for example, K.A. Platt, 'Health and Sanitation', in A.R. Caton (ed.), *The Key of Progress: A Survey of the Status and Conditions of Women in India*, London, Oxford University Press, 1930, pp. 45–79.
3 M. Balfour and R. Young, *The Work of Medical Women in India*, London, Oxford University Press, 1929, p. 182; *A Survey of Medical Missions in India*, Poona, National Christian Council, 1928, pp. 92–3.
4 J. Lowe, *Medical Missions: Their Place and Power*, Edinburgh, Oliphant, Anderson & Ferrier, 1886, p. 204.
5 A.F. Walls, ' "The Heavy Artillery of the Missionary Army": The Domestic Importance of the Nineteenth Century Medical Missionary', in W.J. Shiels (ed.), *The Church and Healing*, Oxford, Blackwell, 1982, p. 288.
6 J. Rutter Williamson, *The Healing of the Nations*, London, Student Volunteer Missionary Union, 1899, p. 92.
7 Balfour and Young, op. cit., p. 76.
8 The concept of 'the double cure', the twofold healing of body and soul, was widely employed in the rhetoric of late nineteenth and early twentieth-century missionary medicine. See, for example, Lowe, op. cit., p. 61; W.J. Wanless, *The Medical Mission: Its Place, Power and Appeal*, Philadelphia, Westminster Press, 1900, p. 39; E.K. Paget, *The Claim of Suffering: A Plea for Medical Missions*, London, Society for the Propagation of the Gospel in Foreign Parts, 1913, p. 115.
9 R. Fletcher Moorshead, *The Appeal of Medical Missions*, Edinburgh, Oliphant, Anderson & Ferrier, 1913, p. 43.
10 Of these 680, 338 were American, 288 British, 27 Canadian, 7 Australian and 20 from Continental Europe; J.S. Dennis, *Christian Missions and Social Progress*, 3 vols, Edinburgh, Oliphant, Anderson & Ferrier, 1899, vol. 2, p. 402.
11 J.S. Dennis, *Centennial Survey of Foreign Missions*, Edinburgh, Oliphant, Anderson & Ferrier, 1902, pp. 113–14, 271.
12 J. Richter, *A History of Missions in India*, Edinburgh, Oliphant, Anderson & Ferrier, 1908, pp. 347, 354.
13 H.P. Beach and B. St John, *World Statistics of Christian Missions*, New York, Foreign Missions Conference of North America, 1916, p. 61.
14 Ibid., p. 96.
15 See, for example, J. Murray, 'Anglican and Protestant Missionary Societies in Great Britain: Their Use of Women as Missionaries from the Late Eighteenth Century to the Late Nineteenth Century', *Exchange*, 1992, vol. 21, pp. 1–28; D. Kirkwood, 'Protestant

Missionary Women: Wives and Spinsters', in F. Bowie, D. Kirkwood and S. Ardener (eds), *Women and Missions: Past and Present*, Oxford, Berg, 1993.

16 H. Callan and S. Ardener (eds), *The Incorporated Wife*, London, Croom Helm, 1984.

17 J. Johnston (ed.), *Report of the Centenary Conference on the Protestant Missions of the World*, London, Nisbet, 2 vols, 1888, vol. 2, p. 157.

18 The phrase 'women's work for women' was commonly used, by European and North American missionary societies and their supporters, to denote the sphere of women missionaries' activities overseas. See, for example, L.A. Flemming (ed.), *Women's Work for Women: Missionaries and Social Change in Asia*, London, Westview Press, 1989.

19 Johnston, op. cit., vol. 2, p. 145.

20 *Statistical Atlas of Christian Missions*, Edinburgh, World Missionary Conference, 1910, p. 63.

21 In 1910 almost 21 per cent of all male missionaries served in India, 20 per cent in China. ibid., pp. 66–9.

22 W. Elmslie, *Medical Missions as illustrated by some letters and notices of the late Dr Elmslie*, (J. Lowe, ed.), Edinburgh, Edinburgh Medical Missionary Society, 1874, p. 191.

23 J. Nair, 'Uncovering the Zenana: Visions of Indian Womanhood in Englishwomen's Writings, 1813–1940', *Journal of Women's History*, 1990, vol. 2, p. 11.

24 J.S. Dennis, *Foreign Missions After A Century*, Edinburgh, Oliphant, Anderson & Ferrier, 1894, pp. 325–6.

25 Elmslie, op. cit., p. 198.

26 Ibid., p. 191.

27 It was widely reported to Western audiences that secluded Indian women would rather die than be treated by a medical man and that even unsecluded women were reluctant to consult male practitioners for treatment of 'diseases peculiar to women'. Rutter Williamson, op. cit., p. 29.

28 Elmslie, op. cit. p. 203.

29 E. Storrow, *Our Indian Sisters*, New York, Fleming H. Revell, n.d., p. 71.

30 Richter, op. cit., p. 329.

31 Fletcher Moorshead, op. cit., pp. 140–1.

32 Dennis, *Centennial Survey*, p. 264.

33 Ibid., p. 207.

34 In 1916, only 16 per cent (122) of all male missionary doctors were stationed in India; 44 per cent (328) were in China; Beach and St John, op. cit., p. 61.

35 In 1916, 30 per cent of all women missionary doctors and 24 per cent of missionary nurses were serving in China; ibid.

36 Balfour and Young, op. cit., p. 14.

37 Elmslie, op. cit., p. 194.

38 Lowe, op. cit., p. 33.

39 Ibid., p. 185.
40 Ibid., p. 188.
41 Ibid., pp. 189, 192, 195.
42 E.T. Fox, *A Missionary Directory for Nurses*, Nottingham, H.B. Saxton, 1908.
43 Fletcher Moorshead, op. cit., p. 155.
44 The number of British missionary nurses working in India rose from 137 in 1905 to 270 in 1910; 'The Training of the Missionary Nurse', *Nursing Journal of India*, 1910, vol. 1, p. 171.
45 J. Muller, 'Some Personal Reminiscences of Work in the Delhi Medical Mission: 1884–1910', *Cambridge Mission to Delhi, Short Papers*, 1910, p. 13, Cambridge Brotherhood Library, Delhi.
46 Ibid., p. 12.
47 Fletcher Moorshead, op. cit., p. 152.
48 W.R. Lambuth, *Medical Missions: The Twofold Task*, New York, Student Volunteer Movement, 1920, p. 151.
49 Paget, op. cit., pp. 87–90.
50 Fletcher Moorshead, op. cit., p. 96.
51 Christian Medical Association of India, Burma and Ceylon, *Tales From The Inns of Healing*, Nagpur, Christian Medical Association of India, Burma and Ceylon, 1942, pp. 148–9.

Chapter 5

Outside the profession: nursing staff on Robben Island, 1846–1910

Harriet Deacon

INTRODUCTION

Traditional histories of nursing in Britain have focused on the professionalization of nursing and the role nursing reformers such as Florence Nightingale and Mrs Bedford Fenwick played in this process. In South Africa, there has been a similar emphasis on the 'progressive' reforms made by Sister Henrietta and her followers in the late nineteenth century. Revisionist historians have now challenged the traditional view which eulogizes the rise of a lily-white nursing profession from the ashes of Sarah Gamp.[1] It is certainly true that the changes in nursing recruitment and training in the last quarter of the nineteenth century affected hospitals profoundly and there were major conflicts with doctors over the growing power of nurses and the administrative changes the new nursing sisters pressed for in the hospitals. But insofar as the introduction of state registration was an important positive influence on the status and material rewards of nursing at all – a matter of some debate – it may have done so at the expense of a patient-centred approach to healing and nurses' independence, creating exploitation, subservience and dependence of nurses.[2]

In accordance with the trend towards problematizing the interpretation of professionalization it has been recognized that an analysis of nursing history may be most usefully approached not as a long haul towards professionalization but as a chapter in labour history. As Christopher Maggs has pointed out, 'nursing is an economic activity' and is closely related to employment markets outside the hospital.[3] In the history of nursing in South Africa the need for such an approach is very evident. Historians have now also begun to examine the relatively neglected fields of mental nursing history (mental nurses were not represented as 'ministering angels' like the Nightingale nurses) and pauper nursing history (pauper nurses continued to be seen as Gamp-like figures) although the major focus remains on the general hospital nurse.[4] It has also been recognized that there are important continuities between the staffing patterns in hospitals of the mid-nineteenth century and the subsequent era of professionalization and registration. In the Cape Colony, racialized and gendered patterns of employment were in place well before the late nineteenth century. These patterns were, and continued to be, influenced by a range of factors such as racism, the state of the local labour market, the kind of patient clientele and the status of the hospital. This chapter examines the process of gendering and racialization within the nursing staff at two institutions, a mental asylum and a leper hospital, situated on Robben Island, between their establishment in 1846 and their closure in 1921 and 1931 respectively.

Shula Marks has spoken of the nursing profession in South Africa as a divided sisterhood – divided along lines of gender, race, class and ethnicity.[5] The division of the profession was cemented at the very beginning of professional nursing, which pushed male and black female nurses out of the general hospitals. But these divisions had their roots in a long history of gendered and racialized employment patterns. In Cape medical institutions of the early nineteenth century, nursing was a low-status task performed by slaves and patients. These posts were gradually filled by working-class British immigrants, a trend which increased as services expanded in the 1850s. The first Nightingale-trained nurses came to the Cape in the 1870s with the Anglican sisterhoods, who had already been active in Cape Town since the 1860s. Once the sisterhoods had taken over general nursing in the 1870s, white nurses were entrenched as the symbol of the profession, embodying its missionary aspects. The sisterhoods dominated general nursing and training until the turn of the century, when they were displaced by their secular trainees. A few black nurses had been employed to nurse in general hospitals as early as the 1850s. But they were specifically excluded from nursing by the early twentieth century, and were only to enter the profession in significant numbers after 1950. Concern about using white nurses for 'degrading tasks' eventually provided the opening for the training and employment of more black nurses in South Africa.[6]

The growing predominance of white, female, trained nursing staff in general hospitals in South Africa was not emulated in all medical institutions. Staffing in the Robben Island leper hospital and mental asylum, which employed a consistently high number of men and untrained nurses in an all-white staff, departed in several respects from trends in general hospitals and also from some of the trends in leper hospitals and asylums on the mainland. Men continued to be employed (although sometimes in lower numbers) in mental asylums, both in Britain and in the colony, after female nurses had taken over in general hospitals. Although white nurses dominated the general hospital and asylum staffs in the colony, black nurses were employed as an 'experiment', at largely black asylums such as Fort Beaufort. Low-status leper nursing was done mainly by black nurses in asylums such as Emjanyana in the Transkei (Eastern Cape) where the patients were all black.[7] And during the early twentieth century an increasing number of female staff were employed in Cape leper hospitals on the mainland.

The particular circumstances of Robben Island, which was isolated and had a poor public reputation, the marginality of leper and mental hospitals, and the colonial situation, all contributed to the production of a pattern of nursing recruitment at Robben Island which was distinctive and conservative. Although Robben Island was certainly an exception to the general trend towards employing white female nurses for white patients and black female nurses for black patients, the Robben Island case study highlights some of the different reasons for gendered and racialized nursing recruitment. In examining the various influences on staffing patterns this chapter begins with an examination of the colonial context of medical provision and then examines employment patterns of nurses during three periods in the history of the Robben Island institutions: the early period, 1846–62, the reforms in the lunatic asylum during the 1860s, and the expansion and reform of the leper hospital in the 1890s.

NURSING HISTORY IN THE COLONIAL CONTEXT

Three features of colonial medical history provide the context for an examination of medical provision at the Cape: the limited role of the state in welfare provision, the strength of the medical profession and the growing influence of racism in shaping colonial society from the mid-nineteenth century. The colonial state was reluctant to provide welfare services at the Cape, in keeping with ideas represented in the English New Poor Law of 1834, and the view that the colony, which had a chronic labour shortage, should support the poor through the provision of employment or private relief. State aid to those who fell on public charity was mainly channelled through gaols and gaol infirmaries or through non-governmental agencies like the churches and private charities. (The Anglican church was later to play an important role in hospital provision by bringing the first Nightingale-trained nurses to the Cape.) But the churches increasingly catered for the welfare needs of their members alone – thus favouring the Afrikaner and English communities. As the colony expanded, however, an infrastructure of mission stations, hospitals, schools and other institutions provided more state-funded services which were often used by the poor. With the extension of the colony eastwards, into territory formerly occupied by independent African groups, medical care in hospitals was also seen as a tool of civilization. Of the seven hospitals in the colony before 1871, four were in the Eastern Cape, where they were built in the 1850s, partly to break the power of traditional African healers.

By the late nineteenth century, and even before, Cape doctors can be seen as 'agents of empire', co-operating closely with the colonial state.[8] Although numerically weak, colonial doctors were in a relatively strong position. The social status of doctors in colonies such as Victoria, for example, was higher than in Britain, and 'regular' practitioners enjoyed government support in Lower Canada through the appointment of Medical Boards, official recognition of medical training and preferential employment.[9,10] In the Cape a medical committee was set up as early as 1807 to regulate practitioners and advise the government on medical matters. 'Regular' doctors enjoyed some degree of preference in appointments to institutional posts, especially in Cape Town. The medical profession only emerged as an organized body in the 1890s but by then, colonial doctors already enjoyed high social status and considerable influence.[11] Secure in their authority, doctors supported early registration of nurses and midwives in 1891. The nurses pressing for registration presented little threat to the doctors' power as they followed the deferential Nightingale model.[12]

Nurses too, were 'agents of empire', and the continuing concern with the type of woman employed as nurse in the colonies testifies to fears, in Britain and abroad, that the wrong sort of nurse would reflect badly on the imperial enterprise. The question of fitness to nurse was tinged with a growing racism by the late nineteenth century, as the right sort of nurse was explicitly represented as white. A major concern, both in India and, by the later nineteenth century in South Africa, was the fear of black hands exerting institutional authority on white bodies.[13] There were, however, contradictory strands in the tale in the earlier part of the century. There was a close identification between blackness and domestic labour, with which nursing was closely associated in Britain until the 1860s, and a definite reluctance on the part of white colonists to engage in menial tasks. By the 1880s, however, respectability, so essential to the reformed nurse, was increasingly seen as a white characteristic, and nursing was dissociated from ordinary domestic labour. At the same time, fears of the black domestic servant as a carrier of disease, especially syphilis, had become a powerful public touchstone, making her unfit to nurse.[14]

THE ROBBEN ISLAND HOSPITALS

The 'General Infirmary' was established on Robben Island by the colonial government in 1846 to house destitute lepers, lunatics and the chronic sick. Immigration and the emancipation of slaves in 1838 brought an increase in the number of destitute people without family or other support networks at the Cape for whom there was felt to be some imperial responsibility. The colonial state stepped into the breach by providing institutions such as Robben Island to control the possible disruptive effects of rapid urbanization in the ex-slave population and to assist those ex-slaves and immigrants who were unable to work or get charitable assistance in Cape Town. The Colonial Secretary, John Montagu, had begun a wide-ranging set of reforms in the early 1840s, partly to reduce the colonial deficit, but more broadly, to re-establish the social hierarchy in the wake of amelioration in the 1820s and the emancipation of slaves.

Montagu centralized and rationalized the colony's institutional network, creating a utilitarian 'pauper economy' based on the idea of reform through labour, and thus the creation of a colonial working class. Convicts, 'domesticated' as workers, were now employed on road and harbour works on the mainland. Lunatics had always been a disruptive influence in the gaols, but this became increasingly problematic within Montagu's new convict system. The chronic sick poor also filled gaol infirmary beds and scarce hospital accommodation without providing the possibility of reform, and lepers were seen as a growing threat at a time of increased mobility and communication. Montagu wanted to reduce the cost of supporting the sick poor and planned the General Infirmary to rationalize and centralize institutional provision for those who presented a threat to society with little chance of reform or usefulness. He therefore removed the now potentially useful and reformable convicts from Robben Island and replaced them with incurably sick paupers.

Until the 1860s the General Infirmary was a custodial institution, both by intent and in practice. As a custodial institution, it was modelled on the 'less eligible' poorhouse and had its colonial origins in the early colonial practice of housing lunatics and the sick poor in gaol infirmaries. It had its institutional justification in Montagu's utilitarian reforms and the acceptance of medical supervision over its chronic inmates. During the 1850s, the population at Robben Island approximated those in British workhouses, which were filling up with the aged and infirm and contained many pauper lunatics who were unable to find places in the new county asylums.[15] The General Infirmary was also similar to the poorhouse in organizational form. There was little differentiation in billeting and care for the lepers, lunatics and chronic sick and very few paid staff in the Infirmary at first – much of the nursing was done by patients themselves.

The balance of patient numbers in the three institutions changed over time, following changing managerial priorities which in turn influenced staffing decisions. Chronic sick patients predominated during the 1850s, lunatics during and after the 1860s, and lepers after 1892. The patients were segregated by gender and type (leper, lunatic, chronic sick) but distinctions were also made on the basis of class, ability to work and, increasingly during the 1870s, race. Most of the patients sent to Robben Island after 1846 came from Cape Town, representatives of a growing number of urban poor. The patients were mostly of Khoi and ex-slave origin, at least initially; an increasing number of white lunatics and chronic sick patients were admitted during the 1860s and 1870s and a greater (although never large) proportion of white lepers entered the leper hospital after the 1890s. The whites who were admitted to Robben Island before the 1890s were mainly poor immigrants from Britain who had failed to make their living in Cape Town. This was the same group from which most of the subordinate staff at Robben Island were recruited.

For some years after the establishment of the Infirmary in 1846 the Island staff was very small, with only six staff members in the institution, besides boatmen.[16] The staff was also characterized by social divisions. Commandant Wolfe, who had run the Island prison for some years, stayed on as the head of the Infirmary for a year, when his role was taken over by the English doctor, John Birtwhistle, who had come as Resident Surgeon in 1846. Birtwhistle was made Surgeon-Superintendent in 1847.[17] Together with the Chaplain (Rev. Lehmann) and the Clerk and storekeeper (David Thompson), who had come from the Somerset Hospital, they formed the upper echelon of the staff, who were a potentially cohesive group. In 1847, a memorialist to government proposed a storekeeper for Robben Island who would 'promote good society' with the Chaplain and the Doctor.[18]

The distinction between the upper and lower levels of staff was reinforced by large discrepancies in pay, as Thompson received £90 a year at the lowest end of the officials' scale while subordinate staff salaries ranged from £6 to £30 per annum.[19] An 'overseer of the sick' tended the male lepers and chronic sick and offloaded stores with the lunatics' aid. The clerk's wife, Mrs Thompson, was appointed to look after the clothing of the female sick, the washing and the leper children.[20] A lunatic keeper and matron came from the Somerset Hospital and a matron was hired for the female chronic sick hospital in 1847. The chronic-sick matron was expected to supervise the washing done by the female lunatics, until a separate post was created by 1858.[21,22] By 1861, after a number of new appointments, for over 300 patients there were still only three male and one female chronic sick attendants, four male and three female lunatic staff (including matrons and keepers), and one male and one female leper attendant (these were patients who were paid a small salary).[23]

Robben Island did not attract staff easily. For doctors the pay was too low to offset the disadvantage of losing private practice in the town.[24] Montagu had struggled to find a doctor willing to go to the Island, and had offered the post to several medical men, but all had refused.[25] Dr Birtwhistle, described in 1853 as having 'a weather-beaten, florid countenance and a quick, sharp, restless eye', was fresh out from England in 1846 with a MRCS qualification (London, 1827).[26,27] He was unmarried, and was virtually unknown in the colony, but after his dismissal in 1855 he returned to England and was made a Fellow of the Royal College of Surgeons in 1856.[28]

The poor public image of the island made recruitment of subordinate staff difficult.[29] Wolfe had written to Montagu in 1844 that:

> it is impossible to prevail on respectable free servants to come to Robben Island. Their answer is; first, if we take service at Robben Island, whenever we leave it and wish to obtain other service, people imagine that, having lived at the island we have either been convicts, or such scamps that we were obliged to go there; second, we are cut off from our wives, families and friends, and have no society or recreation.[30]

The General Infirmary had to compete with local labour markets (especially in domestic service and the police) and nursing work was of low status generally.[31] Private nurses and nannies, usually destitute, elderly or widowed women, were more poorly paid than servants in Cape Town, certainly during the 1850s.[32] And institutional pay was not normally high – British pauper asylums generally paid their attendants less than ordinary servants.[33] Wolfe had paid his personal servant double the going rate in Cape Town, but the General Infirmary did not try to attract people of such calibre.[34] Robben Island chronic sick attendants earned less than ward attendants at Somerset Hospital until 1853 when they got £24 per annum, and lunatic asylum staff were paid less than domestic servants in Cape Town even in 1855.[35,36]

There were hidden attractions of employment at the General Infirmary, however. The more senior posts at Robben Island carried greater responsibility and a higher salary than a position of servant or labourer.[37] Although Robben Island lacked the multiple employment opportunities offered by Cape Town, which allowed many among the working classes to eke out an existence on low salaries, staff could sell their rations, raise pigs and grow vegetables.[38,39] One attendant, O'Brien, disappeared to Cape Town with several patients' money.[40] Robben Island held out the promise of year-round employment with board and lodging, worth about £25 per annum.[41,42] This was essential. Judges has calculated that the minimum monthly income required to support a family of five in Cape Town during the 1830s was £3/8/10.[43] In 1849, the lunatic matron was earning only £1/5/–per month and the gatekeeper (lunatic keeper), £1/10/–per month after two pay rises.[44] It was almost impossible to find people to come to the Island as single domestic servants, but the Island nursing posts, which guaranteed employment and maintenance, held some attractions for the married couple.[45]

Many staff came to the Island because of personal connections. Mrs Young, chronic sick matron between 1849 and 1851, had a son who had been a patient at the General Infirmary since 1846.[46] Mrs Dunbar came from England to stay with her daughter who was Superintendent of Washing on the Island, in 1860 and was soon employed as a lunatic matron.[47] The Simpsons' daughter, Johanna, remained on Robben Island until her death in 1892.[48] Children of employees often took Island posts. The butcher and baker, William Jenkins, employed his son as assistant in the 1850s. Their family had been on the Island since about 1840.[49] After leaving in 1854, Jenkins was to return as a chronic sick patient in 1876.[50] Convalescent patients were often employed at Robben Island, as in British pauper institutions.[51] Joseph Francis, a sailor who was sent to Robben Island as a lunatic in 1853, chose to work in the surf boat for meat and clothes for some time after his recovery before going to take a post on a whaling vessel from Simonstown in 1855.[52] In 1862, two of the male lunatic attendants were convalescent patients.[53] The Infirmary thus acted partly as a workhouse for the staff, providing sheltered employment, with board and lodging, for those who would otherwise be destitute in the town, but without publicly assuming responsibility for the relief of the able-bodied poor.

Female nursing staff at Robben Island before the 1860s were all drawn from the lower ranks of the immigrant servant class, judging pay levels, but it is hard to tell whether they had been involved in paid domestic labour prior to their move to the Island. The mid-century nurse at Robben Island was usually middle-aged and often poorly educated. Jane Rose, chronic sick matron at Robben Island in 1853, could not even write her own name.[54] They were probably in a similar position to the paid nurses in British hospitals and workhouses during the pre-Nightingale era who were middle-aged, generally married and with nursing experience gained in the family.[55] Many of the female staff were the wives of male employees at the Island. Minto specifically advertised in the Cape Town papers for a married couple to take the posts of ward attendant and Superintendent of Washing in 1855, asking for certificates of good character as references.[56] In British Poor Law Infirmaries, the Matron and Master continued to administer the institution until the late nineteenth century.[57] Married couples were often recruited as matron and keeper to British asylums before the mid-century, when the arrangement lost its popularity.[58] At Somerset Hospital and Robben Island, this practice was to continue well into the 1880s.

Male nursing staff were often drawn from the same labour pool that served the police force. For immigrants, the poorest of whom were Irish, public service employment was an attractive option.[59] Many became policemen. Two of the sick attendants at Somerset Hospital in the 1840s were Irish, as were some of the Robben Island staff.[60] James Nutt, who was employed at the Robben Island asylum from 1855 to 1881, had worked as a constable at a convict station for five years previously. After he left the Island, his attempt to set up a canteen in Cape Town failed, as did applications for a post as constable at the Breakwater convict station, and he was finally re-employed as night watchman on the Island in the mid-1880s.[61] His wife remained on the Island as lunatic matron throughout this period. Ralph Harvey was first employed on the surf boat at Robben Island in the 1850s, then as second lunatic keeper and then left the Island to work in the Cape Town Police.[62] A high staff turnover was characteristic of both the General Infirmary and the police force.[63]

Many of the Robben Island staff had also served in the army. The employment of ex-soldiers was commonplace in workhouses and asylums in England in the mid-nineteenth century.[64] In 1853, the assistant lunatic keeper at Robben Island was Alexander Rose, a pensioner from the 91st Regiment.[65] Another ex-soldier was D. Byrne, lunatic keeper, who was dismissed in 1855 for drunkenness, to the dismay of his wife Eleanor who briefly retained her job as chronic sick matron and superintendent of washing.[66] One of the few staff with previous medical experience, John Simpson, a Scot, was employed as ward attendant and surgeryman (dispenser) after pay rises in the mid-1850s. He had been a hospital sergeant of the 25th Regiment of Foot. He died on the Island in 1863 and his wife, employed as a lunatic matron, died there in 1877.

An examination of the social profile of the Robben Island nursing staff in the 1840s and 1850s thus reveals a bias towards employing low-status white immigrant labour. The colonial government seems to have given particular assistance to these British immigrants, who were competing with unskilled black workers (including ex-slaves) in the urban job market. Immigration to South Africa from Britain, which began in earnest in the 1820s, was promoted by government schemes to aid immigration in the period 1848–51, bringing 4,200 settlers, and the colonial government felt some obligation to provide further aid where needed. Certainly, state assistance for the sick poor at Robben Island seems to have been more readily given to immigrants than local blacks after the 1860s. By also providing the Robben Island nursing staff with employment and sometimes care in retirement the colonial state extended special assistance to a group of more physically able but impoverished British immigrants. This helped to reduce the number of poor immigrants who became part of the threatening urban underclass in Cape Town.

THE IMPACT OF ASYLUM REFORMS ON THE NURSING STAFF 1852–70

During the 1850s the custodial approach, which explicitly favoured the Island site as a place of exclusion with the healthy features of fresh air and sea bathing merely an added advantage, began to conflict with the idea that the medical institution should be a site where medical cure could be effected in an environment that stressed return to normality rather than exclusion from it. The Robben Island mental asylum began to attract reformist attention similar to that in Britain and elsewhere which stressed the importance of curing the insane through a humanitarian regime of 'moral management' and 'non-restraint'. In the mid-1850s scandals about mismanagement and cruelty at Robben Island were sparked off by a conflict between the Infirmary's Clerk and Storekeeper and the Surgeon-Superintendent. The issues were taken up by local interests in the Cape Parliament anxious to criticize the Colonial Office as well as by doctors eager to rescue the reputation of their profession. The transition to a curative ethos was to affect the chronic sick and lepers much later. They continued to be nursed by a small number of staff and mobile patients until the 1890s, when the chronic sick were removed to hospitals on the mainland and the notion of a curative 'hospital' for lepers became more popular once bacteriological investigations into the disease had generated some therapeutic optimism.

The colonial government and the Cape medical profession responded to the asylum scandals in the 1850s by blaming first inadequate facilities and staffing, and then the Island site itself. Forced to counter charges of inhumanity and retrogressiveness in their approach towards the insane, but reluctant to expand its welfare operations in the colony, the government preferred to make alterations within the Robben Island asylum rather than responding to calls to remove the institution from the Island altogether. In 1862 they appointed a new Surgeon-Superintendent at the Infirmary, William Edmunds, who began the process of reform in earnest. A crucial part of the reforms, in the absence of any successful pharmaceutical therapies, was the introduction of new nursing procedures under the system of 'moral management', which demanded closer supervision of patients and personal restraint by keepers and seclusion cells rather than the use of handcuffs, chains or 'depletory' (sedative) medicines. Edmunds noted in the annual report for 1863 that attendants were better trained and acted with firmness and decision, using no force or noise.[67]

Edmunds' reforms had a significant impact on the asylum staff. The number of staff at the Infirmary increased dramatically during the 1860s, especially in the lunatic asylum. The total number of staff increased from twenty in 1858 to over fifty in 1871. This meant that by 1871 there were more staff at Robben Island than any other colonial hospital.[68] Pay rises were also given in the early 1860s to attract a 'better class' of attendant.[69] By 1873, Robben Island female asylum nurses earned over three times the salary of a cook or domestic servant in Cape Town, whereas in the early 1850s, they had been earning less than a domestic servant.[70] Because of the high turnover among the nursing staff, a new system of pay increases after every three years' service was introduced in 1862 to encourage staff to stay longer.[71] A group of new asylum staff began to coalesce. In 1868 just under half of the asylum staff had been employed in their posts

for over two years, but only four had been employed before
Edmunds took over. Three-fifths were married to other Island
employees.[72] By 1871, three-fifths had been there for over two
years.[73] (Turnover rates in English asylums averaged 33 per cent
per annum towards the end of the century and were considered
high.)[74]

Edmunds also introduced stricter supervision of staff (through
tell-tale clocks, order books and hierarchical divisions) and better
delineation of staff duties (rules were drawn up in 1866).[75] The
introduction of uniforms in 1871 and 1873 underlined the new
role of staff as symbols of order, discipline and morality.[76,77] In
choosing new staff restrictions were placed on applicants' age
(staff had to be over twenty-five), number of dependants, and
marital status (only single women were recruited from 1871
and single men from 1878).[78,79,80,81] Edmunds felt that employing
unmarried staff would be cheaper, reduce absenteeism for family
reasons and would bring the institution into line with European
asylums.[82] It also allowed tighter control over activities outside
working hours: by 1878 the female attendants had to be in their
quarters by 8 p.m.[83]

In the wave of staff appointments during the 1860s more British
immigrants were employed on the Robben Island asylum staff
but these people were of a higher status in the labour market.
Applications for posts at Robben Island increased to such an
extent that the Surgeon-Superintendent could afford to reject
some with families or drinking problems, and did not have to
advertise.[84] Between 1859 and 1867 over twelve thousand British
immigrants had been brought to the Cape on government
schemes, many of them skilled labourers for the building and
railway schemes of the late 1850s.[85] Most of the immigrants went
to the towns, of which Cape Town was one of the largest. By
1875 immigrant Europeans represented 10 per cent of the colonial
white population.[86] Irish immigrants, often very poor and
unskilled, were reluctant to move to places where there were no
Catholic priests and many would have chosen Robben Island as
a preferable option to moving to distant towns like Port Elizabeth.[87] More Scottish immigrants were taken on as Island staff
during the 1860s than before, in spite of the fact that by 1875
and probably beforehand, there were more Irish than Scottish
immigrants in the Cape.[88] Scottish workers were in great demand
in Cape Town, certainly during the 1860s as they were perceived

to be hardworking and reliable.[89] This may be why the Robben Island asylum was eager and, with higher wages, able to employ them.

The discovery of diamonds in 1867 and gold in 1886 enticed more immigrants to the Cape, but many Island staff were attracted to the diamond fields in the 1870s.[90,91] New staff coming into the more undesirable posts (restricted to the unmarried) were more likely to be Irish. This gave a section of the village the name 'Irishtown', a term which referred to Irish ghettos in British towns and in Cape Town (in the 1840s).[92] By the turn of the century, after conflict between Anglican and Roman Catholic interests in the higher levels of staff and changes in recruitment patterns, the number of Irish among the nursing staff seems to have decreased. But after the initial enthusiasm for reforms in the Island staff during the 1860s and 1870s the attractiveness of Island employment seems to have waned somewhat. In 1881 the Surgeon-Superintendent said that because staff pay was so low they often left to better themselves.[93] This was, of course, partly because these staff were people who had prospects of better employment elsewhere. Some staff left because of the low chance of promotion in the small and isolated institution, or to educate their children.[94,95] There was still a high staff turnover in 1894.[96] Even in the early twentieth century, when pay was higher at Robben Island than at other asylums or leper hospitals, turnover remained fairly high. The pattern was similar to that at the Toronto and Gladesville asylums in colonial Australia and Canada which had a high staff turnover, but staff who were prepared to stay were often employed until their deaths.[97]

The staff at Robben Island received a surprisingly good press in spite of continued doubts about the siting of the asylum on the Island. In contrast, Smith comments that English asylum attendants were often the scapegoats for the failures of the lunacy services.[98] At the Toronto Asylum in colonial Canada, too, officials were never satisfied with the staffing – this would have opened the door for criticism of the moral management system.[99] Whereas the introduction of 'moral management' had produced little in the way of pay rises in British pauper asylums, however, staff pay at the Robben Island asylum had nearly quadrupled by the early 1870s. By 1873, Robben Island female asylum nurses were earning £30 per annum, or three times the salary of a cook or domestic servant in Cape Town, whereas in the 1850s, they had been earning less than a domestic servant.[100] Staff were no longer drawn from the housemaid class, but rather from the ranks of upper domestic servants and the artisan class. At Robben Island the high status of the staff and the positive reception of the 'moral management' reforms there, at least until a more sophisticated regime was offered by the Valkenberg Asylum in 1891, reduced the potential for criticism of the staff. Criticism of the 'moral management' system was deflected on to the Island site and the high proportion of black patients increasingly seen as not amenable to such treatment.

The pattern of employing white staff continued and the employment of a few dark-skinned or 'half-coloured' colonial-born staff was now seen as problematic.[101,102] This was not surprising given that the asylum set out to employ staff of a 'better class' than before and that increasing numbers of patients were white. Race was increasingly linked to class by this time, both in rhetoric and reality. Bickford-Smith has argued that during the 1880s and 1890s, the association of whiteness with respectability led to a move from class exclusivity with ethnic undertones, towards a more racially oriented segregationism.[103] Holden has suggested that the concern with class so evident in discourses about nursing recruitment in Britain was even more evident in the colonial situation 'because of the need to maintain distance from, and ideas of superiority to, the native races'.[104] A central issue in 'moral management' was staff character, and the force of example. In Indian asylums, as early as the 1850s, Indian staff had been thought to lack the 'moral and physical courage' and 'tact' necessary to implement a regime of kindness and control without mechanical restraint.[105] Such considerations, and a reluctance to provide black staff for the increasing number of middle-class white patients at the Island asylum, meant that the asylum reforms entrenched the racist employment practices evident in the early years of the General Infirmary. By the 1900s, it was openly proclaimed to be essential to have white asylum nurses, and any suspiciously dark applicants were investigated.

The asylum was now increasingly differentiated, both in organizational and architectural terms, from the hospital model and from the other Robben Island institutions. The pattern of employing male attendants was continued at a time when female nurses (the sisterhoods) were beginning to dominate in general hospitals in the colony. The strength of male attendants became ever more important with the reduction in the use of mechanical restraints. Men were also important as examples of masculinity, to resocialize male patients and to take part in 'male' activities like cricket that were part of the rehabilitative programme in the asylum. By the 1890s, when Robben Island began to take more criminal patients, men were particularly valued as custodians of the dangerous insane.

THE IMPACT OF LEPER HOSPITAL REFORMS ON STAFFING AFTER 1892

By 1892 the perception of leprosy as a black disease, and growing concern about it spreading in the colony, particularly to whites, prompted very harsh legislation to enforce the segregation of all medically-certified lepers in institutions such as Robben Island. Before this, the only lepers who had been unfortunate enough to live on the Island were destitute and friendless, and mainly black. Now, for the first time, lepers were to outnumber all the other groups on the Island, and they were to include a significant proportion of whites. The issues of inadequate provision for certain patients within institutions and later, wrongful confinement, were to figure large in the opposition to segregation. There was considerable, well-articulated opposition voiced by the lepers at Robben Island to the new dispensation. In 1892 they wrote petitions to the Queen, in 1895 they burned down one of the wards, and in the early twentieth century, they marched in protest from their segregated quarters towards the village or the offices a number of times.

But one of the most striking protests, in 1892, was directed partly against a group of trained white nurses. In 1891 Surgeon-Superintendent Dixon had complained that:

> the establishment of a system of male ward attendants for the Leper Hospitals is to be deprecated. The work is such, as falls essentially within the sphere of nursing, and can only be efficiently performed, by persons conversant with the routine of a well-ordered hospital.[106]

As Dr Impey explained later, ordinary nurses would fear to nurse lepers – only 'surgical nurses' who took a great interest in their work could be recruited.[107] Eight trained female nurses were employed during 1892 to nurse male lepers in Pavilion No. 1, the 'hospital'. Four of them were Nightingale-trained English nurses who had been brought out to the colony by Sister Henrietta of Kimberley Hospital, some of the others were from the All Saints' nursing sisterhood in Cape Town which had agreed in 1891 to provide nurses for the Island.[108,109] But in September 1892, when the male lepers revolted against the restrictions on the Island, these nurses were a particular target. The lepers threatened to rape the nurses and other white women in the village if they were not allowed access to the female lepers, and to strike the nurses with their crutches.[110] They objected to the 'hospital' practices of the nurses, which included frequent washing and dressing of ulcers, being woken at 6 a.m. and prevented from lying on their beds after they had been made in the morning.[111,112] A kindly visitor from the Sufferers' Aid Society commented, 'The nurses, it seems, looked upon the institution more in the light of a hospital, whereas it is the home of these people.'[113]

Rather short-sightedly, the Island chaplain commented at the beginning of 1893:

> It is much to be wished that the female [lepers] may before long have the benefit of scientific nursing, which has done so much to increase the comfort of the men.[114]

For the nurses, working shifts from 6:30 a.m. to 5 p.m. without weekends or holidays off, at 'repulsive and dangerous' work with recalcitrant patients and little incentive of cure, the isolated Island was not a place which encouraged them to perform as 'ministering angels' for long.[115,116] By the end of 1893, there were only two of the nurses left. The 'Kimberley nurses', probably Sister Henrietta's recruits, all resigned after a dispute with their matron in 1893.[117] Dr Impey, the new Surgeon-Superintendent, complained that the nurses had been more difficult to manage than the patients, as they first conflicted with the male lepers and then with their superiors. These women 'were not to be trusted at all', he said, as they had been employed on the basis of testimonials rather than colonial references.[118] The two remaining nurses, 'old [and untrained] hands', served the male hospital wards and four patients were employed, at some saving, to dress sores in place of each of the other nurses.[119]

Untrained white female nurses were employed for the female lepers in 1895, with no averse results. Indeed they were seen as important in preventing discontent and managing rebellious situations.[120] In 1900 the Commissioner suggested cautiously that a female nurse should again be employed for the male lepers:

> the seriously ill and the dying should [not] be entirely without the attention that only a woman can give.... Of course, to have the entire staff composed of nurses as was once tried here in the male wards was ridiculous, and naturally ended in a fiasco.[121]

Although they may have wanted to employ more female nurses, fear of patient insurrection stopped them. It was only during the 1920s that the proportion of male staff in the leper wards was finally to drop.[122]

By the 1890s mainland doctors were vigorously promoting the employment of trained female nurses in hospitals. One complained in the *South African Medical Journal* about 'pirate nurses' in the hospitals who contradicted the doctors, and annoyed the patients. '[I]f a nurse is a nurse she should be a trained nurse', said another.[123] Recruitment of trained nurses relied heavily on immigrant nurses because there were no training institutions for general nursing staff at the Cape until the mid-1880s. Since the Crimean War, there had been a long tradition of British nurses working overseas, a practice which allowed women to travel and to earn more than they would at home.[124] Some British-trained nurses applied for jobs at colonial institutions directly, while others were recruited from asylum jobs in Britain.[125,126] The Colonial Nursing Association (CNA) in England helped to place others with colonial institutions.[127] The CNA had been founded in 1895 to send European nurses to government hospitals in the Empire.

It was difficult to employ trained nurses at Robben Island, however. The growth in the number of hospitals (partially state-funded, partially public-funded) at the Cape during the latter half of the nineteenth century increased the demand for trained nurses on the mainland. In 1901 a British nurse working in China wished to take advantage of the temperate climate at the Cape and was told that there was a 'certain demand' for nurses in the colony.[128] But it was seldom that such people chose to come to Robben Island unless they found the idea of leper nursing romantic. Annie Steele, for example, applied from London in 1904, wanting to be a leper nurse.[129] The difficulty of recruiting trained nurses for the female leper wards at Robben Island meant that previous hospital

training was not insisted upon.[130] None of the applicants for the
post of leper Matron in 1900, for example, had had any nursing
training.[131] The All Saints' Sisters were the only significant body
of trained nurses to come to the Island; they arrived to look after
the leper children in 1910. Even then, this only occurred after they
had been marginalized from hospital work on the mainland.[132]

After the removal of most non-criminal white 'lunatic' patients
during the course of the 1890s the Robben Island asylum had
considerable difficulty attracting trained mental nurses as well.
Asylum staff had been able to take a qualifying examination from
the British Medico-Psychological Association (MPA) from 1891
and could thereafter be registered in the colony as trained asylum
attendants and nurses, but between 1891 and 1916 only thirty-
one mental nurses were registered altogether at the Cape, compared to 1,024 general nurses.[133] Most of the trained mental
nurses, nearly two-thirds of whom were men, were snapped up
by the Grahamstown and Valkenberg asylums which catered for
white patients. Very few of the Robben Island asylum staff had
taken the examination and none were registered before 1910.
Two of the Robben Island doctors gave lectures to the nursing
staff for the MPA examination in 1896, but neither of the two
eligible nurses sat the exam.[134] In the following year the only
training programmes for asylum staff in the colony were lectures
held at the Port Alfred, Valkenberg and Grahamstown asylums.
The Robben Island staff had to be satisfied with 'Ambulance
lectures' on first aid.[135] Proper lectures were given in 1904, but
they were not compulsory, in spite of the hope expressed by the
asylum doctors that all Robben Island staff would sit the MPA
exam. Dr Moon complained that asylum nurses were still very
hard to find, mostly 'raw' and too young for the job and likely
to leave soon to get married or to nurse relatives.[136]

CONCLUSIONS

The early racialization of employment in the Robben Island hospitals (and in other Cape hospitals like the Somerset Hospital) is
an important precursor to the more widespread patterns of racist
hospital employment after the arrival of trained Nightingale
nurses in the 1870s. White nurses or attendants were initially
favoured for sheltered employment on the Island because government felt some responsibility for them. During the 1860s better-

class whites were employed in the reformed asylum because they were seen as more respectable and therefore better attendants for the insane. Darker-skinned staff were now explicitly shunned. By the early twentieth century, black nursing staff were no longer employed in colonial hospitals on the mainland, except where these catered largely for black patients. Although Robben Island now had a majority of black patients, by 1913 the practice of employing only whites on the Island staff was a 'long-standing arrangement'.[137] This 'arrangement' depended in part on the presence of a large body of relatively mobile patients, the 'lunatics', who provided labour for menial tasks within the institutions and a small convict station which provided additional manual labourers. As residential segregation became the norm in Cape Town by the early twentieth century, it was inconceivable too that the small village on Robben Island could house both black and white employees.

Men retained their importance as attendants in the asylum on Robben Island as in other asylums, but men also retained their position as leper attendants at Robben Island because of patient opposition to trained female nurses which had become an issue in 1892. Increasing emphasis on the custodial role of the institution, the predominance of criminal or dangerous (and mainly black) lunatics and of a large number of recalcitrant lepers helped to justify the employment of male attendants. Although Robben Island tried to attract trained staff for both the leper and the lunatic institutions as they tried to present themselves as 'hospitals', it was unable to attract trained nurses in any numbers. The staff was large because of the security needed to control the sometimes rebellious lepers and often dangerous 'lunatics'. With the emphasis on control, a large number of Leper Police were employed on the Island from 1895. In 1920, as one of six leper institutions in the Union, Robben Island accounted for one third of the total staff numbers.[138] Although many of the Robben Island nursing staff were without formal training, its reliance on white males, whose salaries had to reflect their high social status, made the Robben Island leper hospital and lunatic asylum very expensive to run, a factor which contributed towards its closure in 1931.[139]

The public image of Robben Island also affected its staffing patterns. The 'moral management' reforms of the 1860s brought a better class of white nursing staff to Robben Island than were attracted to British pauper asylums, and indeed many colonial asylums, partly because of strong central government control over the Robben Island asylum and the willingness to spend considerable effort and money in modernizing the only colonial asylum. The history of the Robben Island site as a place of imprisonment and banishment and the mismanagement scandals of the 1850s meant that the reform effort had to be meticulous. But the poor public image of the site did not fade and contributed to the marginalization of the Island institutions as the expanding mainland hospitals and asylums became the focus of colonial modernization. The continued employment of unregistered nursing staff without formal training was thus particularly evident at Robben Island.

The distinctive makeup of the Robben Island nursing staff was the result of several features of the colonial and institutional framework in which it operated: immigration and government 'responsibility', racism, racialized employment patterns, the urban labour market in the colony, the peculiarities of an island site and the poor public image of Robben Island. While some of these factors are specific to the Robben Island case, others are not. The continuing role of untrained nurses indicates the importance of conceptualizing nursing history beyond the bounds of the nursing profession. Historians must also look more closely at various influences on patterns of employment which meant that Robben Island and other institutions did not follow the general trend in late nineteenth- and early twentieth-century South Africa towards white trained female nurses for white patients and increasingly, black female nurses for black patients.

NOTES

1 C. Davies (ed.), *Rewriting Nursing History*, London, Croom Helm, 1980 and C. Maggs (ed.), *Nursing History: the State of the Art*, London, Croom Helm, 1987.
2 Boston Nurses Group, Hawker and Woods cited in C. Maggs, 'Introduction' in C. Maggs (ed.), op. cit., pp. 4–5.
3 C. Maggs, 'Profit and loss and the hospital nurse' in C. Maggs (ed.), op. cit., p. 176.
4 P. Nolan, *A History of Mental Health Nursing*, London, Chapman and Hall, 1993.
5 S. Marks, *Divided Sisterhood: the Nursing Profession and the Making of Apartheid in South Africa*, London, Macmillan, 1994.

6 'Work of the nurses', *Cape Times*, 16 March 1911 and 'Native nurses in hospitals', *South African News*, 7 May 1913.

7 Annual report on Fort Beaufort Asylum for 1895, *Cape Parliamentary Papers* (CPP), G27–1896, pp. 17–18.

8 E. van Heyningen, 'Agents of Empire: the medical profession in the Cape Colony, 1880–1910', *Medical History*, 1989, vol. 33, p. 450.

9 K.S. Inglis, *Hospital and Community*, Melbourne, Melbourne University Press, 1985, p. 28.

10 G. Bilson, 'Public health and the medical profession in nineteenth-century Canada' in R. MacLeod and M. Lewis (eds), *Disease, Medicine and Empire*, London, Routledge, 1988, p. 158.

11 Van Heyningen, op. cit., p. 462.

12 Marks, op. cit., p. 113–14.

13 W. Ernst, *Mad Tales from the Raj*, London, Routledge, 1991, p. 155; and Marks, op. cit., p. 78.

14 Reports of Civil Commissioners, Resident Magistrates and District Surgeons for 1882, Cape Parliamentary Papers, G91–1883 and Reports of District Surgeons for 1883, Cape Parliamentary Papers, G67–1884.

15 M.A. Crowther, *The Workhouse System*, London, Methuen, 1981, p. 3; G. Rivett, *The Development of the London Hospital System 1823–1982*, London, King Edward's Hospital Fund for London, 1986, p. 63.

16 *Cape of Good Hope Blue Book for 1846*, pp. 176–77.

17 Memorial of Birtwhistle, Jan. 1846, Cape Archives in Cape Town (CA), Memorials received by Colonial Office (CO), CO 4028, doc.78; Montagu to Medical Committee, 15 Feb. 1846, Cape Archives, Medical Committee, Minutes of Proceedings 1842–1848, MC 3.

18 Memorial of Juritz, 23 Feb. 1847, Cape Archives, Memorials received by Colonial Office, CO 4033, doc.131.

19 Birtwhistle to Montagu, 16 Dec. 1848, Cape Archives, Robben Island Papers, Letterbook, RI 1.

20 Wolfe to Montagu, 3 Apr. 1846, Cape Archives, Letters received by Colonial Office on medical matters 1831–46, CO 4372.

21 Wolfe to Montagu, 8 Dec. 1846, Cape Archives, Letters received by Colonial Office on medical matters 1831–46, CO 4372.

22 Eleanor Byrne to Colonial Secretary, 27 Jan. 1855, Cape Archives, Letters received by Colonial Office, CO 659.

23 Dr Minto, Minutes of evidence, Commission of Inquiry into Robben Island, 1861–2, Cape Parliamentary Papers, G31–1862, pp. 3, 6.

24 Debates in Parliament, 27 March 1855, Cape Archives, CCP 3/2/2, p. 138.

25 Two of the refusals were: Memorial of Gill, n.d. 1845, Cape Archives, Memorials received by Colonial Office, CO 4025 (196) and Memorial of Pawle, n.d. 1845, Cape Archives, Memorials received by Colonial Office, CO 4026 (475).

26 Charles Bell, Addendum to Report, Inquiry of 1853, Papers relating

to the Select Committee of 1854, Cape Parliamentary Papers, A37–1855, p. 65.

27 Medical Committee to Montagu, 28 Feb. 1846, Cape Archives, Medical Committee: Minutes of proceedings 1842–1848, MC 3.

28 On his FRCS, see Sir D'Arcy Power and W.G. Spencer (eds), *Plarr's Lives of the Fellows of the Royal College of Surgeons of England*, vol. 1, Bristol, J. Wright, 1930, p. 104. The FRCS was granted by examination after 1843 to candidates, who among other things, showed 'good character' and had 'given satisfactory evidence of efficiency' in hospital and private practice (Z. Cope, *The Royal College of Surgeons of England: a History*, London, Anthony Blond, 1959, pp. 72–4).

29 This continued into the 1860s, see Debates in Parliament, 3 Dec. 1866, Cape Archives, CCP 3/2/3, p. 45.

30 Wolfe to Montagu, 6 Jan. 1844 in Great Britain, 'Papers respecting a plan for improving the discipline of convicts at the Cape of Good Hope, received during the years 1843 and 1844', *Accounts and Papers*, 1847, XLVIII, p. 455.

31 The earnings of a wet nurse in Cape Town during the 1830s, £1/17/6 per month, were comparable to those of a lower servant (L.A. Rushby, 'The Cape and immigration, 1839–1854', unpublished BA (Hons) thesis, University of Cape Town, 1983, p. 25).

32 See for example, the Minutes of the Ladies' Benevolent Society, 5 Aug. 1857 and 1 Apr. 1868, Cape Archives, Dutch Reformed Church Papers, V3 2/1.

33 D.J. Mellett, *The Prerogative of Asylumdom: Social, Cultural and Administrative Aspects of the Institutional Treatment of the Insane in Nineteenth-Century Britain*, New York, Garland, 1982, p. 42.

34 Wolfe to Montagu, 6 Jan. 1844 in Great Britain, op. cit., p. 455.

35 Birtwhistle to Montagu, 27 August 1853, Cape Archives, Robben Island Papers, Letterbook, RI 1.

36 Medical Committee to Colonial Secretary, 19 May 1855 in Select Committee of 1855, Cape Parliamentary Papers, A9–1855, p. 4.

37 The overseer of sick and his wife, who superintended washing and mending, together earned £50 p.a. on Robben Island in 1848 (£4/3/4 per month or £2/1/10 each) (Birtwhistle to Montagu, 16 Dec. 1848, Cape Archives, Robben Island Papers, Letterbook, RI 1). In Cape Town during the 1830s, a labourer earned only £1/16/- per month (£21/12/- p.a.), as did the lowest domestic servant. But some servants could earn almost double this amount (S. Judges, 'Poverty, living conditions and social relations – aspects of life in Cape Town in the 1830s', unpublished MA thesis, University of Cape Town, 1977, p. 10).

38 Judges, op. cit., p. 21.

39 Report, Commission of 1861–2, Cape Parliamentary Papers, G31–1862, p. xiv.

40 Birtwhistle to Montagu, 21 Feb. 1853, Cape Archives, Robben Island Papers, Letterbook, RI 1.

41 Birtwhistle to Montagu, 18 Dec. 1848, Cape Archives, Robben Island Papers, Letterbook, RI1.
42 Birtwhistle to Montagu, 28 Jan. 1850, Cape Archives, Robben Island Papers, Letterbook, RI 1. This was equivalent to £2/1/8 a month.
43 Judges, op. cit., p. 3.
44 Their salaries were £15 and £18 p.a. respectively (Birtwhistle to Montagu, 19 Oct. 1849 and 3 Jan. 1849, Cape Archives, Robben Island Papers, Letterbook, RI 1).
45 Wolfe to Montagu, 6 Jan. 1844 in Great Britain, op. cit., p. 455.
46 Young, Minutes of Evidence, Inquiry of 1852, Papers relating to the Select Committee of 1854, Cape Parliamentary Papers, A37–1855, p. 20.
47 Mrs Dunbar, Minutes of evidence, Commission of 1861–2, Cape Parliamentary Papers, G31–1862, p. 199.
48 M. Coetzee, G. Webber et al., Robben Island cemeteries recording project of the Western Cape Branch of the Genealogical Society of South Africa, Cape Town, Western Cape Genealogical Society, 1993, p. 20.
49 Mrs Jenkins, Minutes of evidence, Inquiry of 1853, Papers relating to the Select Committee of 1854, Cape Parliamentary Papers, A37–1855, p. 107.
50 Chaplain's Diary, 25 Jan. 1876, Johannesburg, University of Witwatersrand Manuscript Collection (UWMC), AB 1162/G3.
51 L. Smith, 'Behind closed doors: lunatic asylum keepers, 1800–60', Social History of Medicine, 1988, vol. 1, no. 3, p. 308.
52 Birtwhistle to Secretary to Government, 5 March 1855, Cape Archives, Letters received by Colonial Office, CO 659.
53 Minto to Colonial Secretary, 27 May 1862, Cape Archives, Letters received by Colonial Office, CO 797.
54 Mrs Rose, Minutes of evidence, Inquiry of 1853, Papers relating to the Select Committee of 1854, Cape Parliamentary Papers, A37–1855, p. 76.
55 B. Abel-Smith, A History of the Nursing Profession, London, Heinemann, 1960, p. 4.
56 Minto to Colonial Secretary, 2 Oct. 1855, Cape Archives, Robben Island Papers, Letterbook, RI 1.
57 R. White, Social Change and the Development of the Nursing Profession: a Study of the Poor Law Nursing Service 1848–1948, London, Henry Kimpton, 1978, pp. 88–9.
58 A. Walk, 'The history of mental nursing', Journal of Mental Science, 1961, vol. 107, p. 6.
59 Judges, op. cit., pp. 148–9.
60 Judges, op. cit., p. 150.
61 Memorial of Nutt, 6 Feb. 1884, Cape Archives, Memorials received by Colonial Office, CO 4243 (N4); Parson to Webb, 25 Feb. 1884, Cape Archives, Letters received by the Breakwater Prison 1881–1885, PBW 2; Nutt, Minutes of evidence, Commission of 1894–5, Cape Parliamentary Papers, G10–1894, p. 327.

62 Harvey, Minutes of evidence, Inquiry of 1852, Papers relating to the Select Committee of 1854, Cape Parliamentary Papers, A37–1855, p. 17.

63 Constables in the Cape Town Police were paid a minimum, at £45 p.a. (£3/15/- p.m.), but a pay increase to £52 p.a. in 1846 stabilized the force somewhat. Nevertheless, turnover was high (K. Elks, 'Crime, community and police in Cape Town, 1825–1850', unpublished MA thesis, University of Cape Town, 1986, pp. 30–1).

64 Mellett, op. cit., p. 42.

65 Memo from Jane Rose to Lieut-Governor, Inquiry of 1853, Papers relating to the Select Committee of 1854, Cape Parliamentary Papers, A37–1855, p. 98.

66 Memorial of Byrne, 23 Feb. 1855, Cape Archives, Memorials received by Colonial Office, CO 4078, doc. B96; E. Byrne to Colonial Secretary, 27 Jan. 1855, Cape Archives, Letters received by Colonial Office, CO 659.

67 Annual Report on Robben Island for 1863, Cape Parliamentary Papers, G3–1864, p. 4.

68 *Cape of Good Hope Blue Book for 1871*, pp. Q78–9.

69 Edmunds to Colonial Secretary, 10 Aug. 1864, Cape Archives, Letters received by Colonial Office, CO 827.

70 Annual report for 1916–1918, Union Parliamentary Papers (UPP), UG31–1920, p. 18; The salary of a black cook and general servant, Catherine, was 18/- p.m. in 1871 (Records of criminal cases, 1 Feb. 1871, Cape Archives, Cape Town Municipality, 1/CT 6/51).

71 *Cape of Good Hope Blue Book for 1860*, pp. Q130–2.

72 Annual report on Robben Island for 1868, Cape Parliamentary Papers, G2–1869, p. 44.

73 Edmunds to Quin, Appendix to Select Committee of 1871, Cape Parliamentary Papers, A3–1871, p. xix.

74 Mercier cited in D. Mellett, op. cit., p. 42.

75 Report of Colonial Medical Committee on inspection of Robben Island, 2 July 1869 in Annual Report on Robben Island for 1868, Cape Parliamentary Papers, G2–1869, p. 47.

76 Dr Biccard to Colonial Secretary, 15 Feb. 1873, Cape Archives, Letters received by the Colonial Office, CO 972.

77 M. Dean and G. Bolton, 'The administration of poverty and the development of nursing practice in nineteenth-century England' in C. Davies (ed.), op. cit., p. 88.

78 Dr Edmunds to Colonial Secretary, 8 June 1869, Cape Archives, Letters received by the Colonial Office, CO 910.

79 Memorial of Sophia Kelly, 20 May 1869, Cape Archives, Memorials received by the Colonial Office, CO 4157 (143). Memorial of Mrs Ormeon, 11 Dec. 1871, Cape Archives, Memorials received by the Colonial Office, CO 4169 (O18).

80 Dr Edmunds to Colonial Secretary, 8 June 1869, Cape Archives, Letters received by the Colonial Office, CO 910. The plan was implemented in 1871.

81 Dr Landsberg to Colonial Secretary, Report of the Colonial Medi-

cal Committee, 4 Jan. 1878, Letters received by the Colonial Office, CO 1067.

82 Dr Edmunds to Colonial Secretary, 8 June 1869, Cape Archives, Letters received by the Colonial Office, CO 910.

83 Chaplain's diary, 5 Mar. 1878, University of the Witwatersrand manuscripts collection (WMC), William Cullen Library, University of the Witwatersrand, Johannesburg, AB 1162.

84 Edmunds to Quin, Appendix to Select Committee of 1871, Cape Parliamentary Papers, A3–1871, p. xix.

85 E. Bull, *Aided Immigration from Britain to South Africa 1857–1867*, Pretoria, Human Sciences Research Council, 1991, pp. 6, 11–12.

86 Census of the Cape Colony for 1891, Cape Parliamentary Papers, G6–1892, p. xxxiii.

87 Bull, op. cit., pp. 41–2.

88 Census of the Cape Colony for 1891, Cape Parliamentary Papers, G6–1892, p. xxxii.

89 Bull, op. cit., p. 41.

90 Bull, op. cit., pp. 13, 17.

91 Chaplain's diary, Report for 1870, notes that the mission school has been much reduced by the removal of several families from the Island and the introduction of single attendants.

92 Judges, op. cit., p. 148.

93 Biccard to Under Colonial Secretary, 28 Feb. 1881, Cape Archives, Letters received by Colonial Office, CO 1162.

94 Biccard to Under Colonial Secretary, 12 Jan. 1881, Cape Archives, Letters received by Colonial Office, CO 1162.

95 Memorial of Widow Kane, 9 Oct. 1860, Cape Archives, Memorials received, CO 4114 (256).

96 Minutes of evidence, Leprosy Commission, Cape Parliamentary Papers, G10–1894, p. 287.

97 W. Mitchinson, 'The Toronto and Gladesville asylums: humane alternatives for the insane in Canada and Australia?', *Bulletin of the History of Medicine*, 1989, vol. 63, p. 68.

98 L.D. Smith, 'Behind closed doors: lunatic asylum keepers, 1800–60', *Social History of Medicine*, 1988, vol. 1, no. 3, p. 327.

99 Mitchinson, op. cit., p. 67.

100 The salary of the black cook and general servant, Catherine, was 18/- per month in 1871. Records of criminal cases, 1 Feb. 1871, Cape Archives, Papers of the Cape Town Resident Magistrate, 1/CT 6/51.

101 Chaplain's diary, 16 Sept. 1885 and 16 Oct. 1885, UWMC, AB 1162.

102 Memorial of Mary King, 3 May 1888, Memorials received by the Colonial Office, CO 4264 (K11). Mary King complains that a 'half-coloured girl' had been employed in her stead.

103 V. Bickford-Smith, *Ethnic Pride and Racial Prejudice in Victorian Cape Town: Group Identity and Social Practice, 1875–1902*, Cambridge, Cambridge University Press, 1995, p. 117.

104 P. Holden, 'Colonial sisters: nurses in Uganda', in P. Holden and J. Littlewood (eds), *Anthropology and Nursing*, London, Routledge, 1991, p. 69.
105 Ernst, op. cit., p. 154.
106 Dr Dixon to Under Colonial Secretary, 27 Aug. 1891, Cape Archives, Letters received by the Colonial Office, CO 1498.
107 Dr Impey, Minutes of evidence, Leprosy Commission, Cape Parliamentary Papers, G10–1894, p. 355.
108 Dr Impey, Minutes of evidence, Leprosy Commission, Cape Parliamentary Papers, G10–1894, p. 355.
109 Dr Dixon to Under Colonial Secretary, n.d. Aug. 1891, Cape Archives, Letters received by the Colonial Office, CO 1498.
110 The male lepers had long been allowed some social intercourse with the female lepers within the institution and the restriction of these privileges in the early 1890s had caused some dissatisfaction.
111 Dr Impey, Minutes of evidence, Leprosy Commission, Cape Parliamentary Papers, G10–1894, p. 355.
112 Mrs St Leger, Minutes of evidence, Leprosy Commission, Cape Parliamentary Papers, G10–1894, p. 298.
113 Mrs St Leger, Minutes of evidence, Leprosy Commission, Cape Parliamentary Papers, G10–1894, p. 298.
114 Revd Watkins, Draft Chaplain's report for 1892, Impey to Under Colonial Secretary, 14 Jan. 1893, Cape Archives, Letters received by the Colonial Office, CO 1586.
115 Under Colonial Secretary to Dr Impey, 29 Dec. 1892, Cape Archives, Letters received by the Colonial Office, CO 1586.
116 Dr Impey, Minutes of evidence, Leprosy Commission, Cape Parliamentary Papers, G10–1894, p. 355.
117 Dr Todd, Minutes of evidence, Leprosy Commission, Cape Parliamentary Papers, G10–1894, p. 229.
118 Dr Impey, Minutes of evidence, Leprosy Commission, Cape Parliamentary Papers, G10–1894, p. 355.
119 Annual report on Robben Island for 1893, Cape Parliamentary Papers, G24–1894, pp. 94–5.
120 Annual report on Robben Island for 1896, Cape Parliamentary Papers, G20–1897, p. 95.
121 Annual report on Robben Island for 1900, Cape Parliamentary Papers, G41–1901, p. 112.
122 Annual report on Robben Island for 1922, Union Parliamentary Papers (UPP), UG9–1924, p. 297 and Annual report on Robben Island for 1926–7, UPP, UG35–1927, p. 22.
123 Letters, *South African Medical Journal*, Apr. 1896, pp. 340–2.
124 Holden, op. cit., p. 68.
125 Under Colonial Secretary to Medical Superintendent at Port Alfred Asylum, 5 June 1903, Cape Archives, Correspondence received by Health Branch, CO 7379, Folio 300.
126 W.R. MacPhail of Derby Borough County Asylum in England to Agent General in Cape Town, 29 May 1903, Cape Archives, Correspondence received by Health Branch, CO 7379, Folio 300.

127 A. Lyttelton (Downing Street) to Colonial Secretary, 15 Feb. 1904, Cape Archives, Correspondence received by Health Branch, CO 7379, Folio 300.

128 Miss M.J. Davies (China) to Under Colonial Secretary, 26 Aug. 1901, Cape Archives, Correspondence received by Health Branch, CO 7379, Folio 300.

129 A. Steele (London) to Colonial Secretary, 15 Apr. 1904, Cape Archives, Correspondence received by Health Branch, CO 7596, Folio 959.

130 Under Colonial Secretary to E.A. Wells (a nurse in England), 5 Aug. 1903, Cape Archives, Correspondence received by Health Branch, CO 7379, Folio 300.

131 Commissioner Piers to Under Colonial Secretary, 21 Aug. 1900, Cape Archives, Correspondence received by Health Branch, CO 7596, Folio 959.

132 Commissioner Jackson to Under Colonial Secretary, 29 Oct. 1901, Cape Archives, Robben Island letterbooks, RI 61.

133 Annual report on Robben Island for 1916, UPP, UG50–1916, p. 2.

134 Annual report on Robben Island for 1896, Cape Parliamentary Papers, G20–1897, p. 101.

135 Extract from Dr Dodds' report on Asylums for 1897, Correspondence received by Health Branch, CO 7514, Folio 645.

136 Memorandum of Dr Moon, 26 Dec. 1904, Cape Archives, Correspondence received by Health Branch, CO 7966, Folio G9d.

137 Annual report on Robben Island for 1913, UPP, UG24–1913, p. 6.

138 Annual report on Robben Island for 1920, UPP, UG8–1922, p. 383.

139 Annual report on Robben Island for 1922, UPP, UG9–1922, p. 297.

Chapter 6

Convicts and care giving in colonial Australia, 1788–1868

Angela Cushing

INTRODUCTION

There has been little attempt to examine convicts and care giving in colonial Australia from a nursing perspective for the period between settlement in 1788 and the introduction of what is known as 'female nursing' in 1868. The notable exception to the dearth of material is Bartz Schultz's *A Tapestry of Service*; however, the study's main shortcoming, as the author acknowledges, is the absence of critical analysis and interpretation.[1] Rather it is a chronological narrative about people, events and institutions with little effort to investigate these in the light of their respective influence on the development of health care and services.[2] This chapter attempts to redress some of the omissions. The account does so in that it incorporates relevant observations from other scholars, offering comment about historiographical concerns crucial to an understanding of the status and image of the convict worker in British and colonial society, particular attention being given to convict women. Thus in so doing it elaborates upon points made by Schultz and analyses the evolution of health care and the emergence of female nursing.

It should be noted that the terms 'care giving' and 'care giver' are employed loosely to denote the activities in which the attendants charged with looking after the poor, the ill and infirm were engaged. To distinguish these terms from that of 'nurse' assists us in appreciating the significance of the changes in caring practice that the introduction of Nightingale nursing brought *vis-à-vis* the trained nurse and the untrained care attendant. While the historical record seems to suggest that the presence of compassion and empathy were not so frequently demonstrated by the early care givers and the equipment and facilities crude and basic, such evidence cannot be accepted at face value. Facilities in colonial Australia were established for the purpose of providing shelter and attendants were present to give attention to those who became patients. Thus it is not unreasonable to refer to those involved in the embryonic beginnings of Australia's health service in terms of 'care givers'.

Various synonyms are employed in the sources to describe the care givers.[3] Female attendants, up to about the 1830s, are usually referred to as either female servants, female domestics or nurses and less frequently by personal name. Later, as care giving became more structured and institutionalized the same terms were used while others were added to the vocabulary. For instance, titles such as wardsmaids, head nurse, under nurse and matron appear. Male care givers, in the early period, are referred to as either attendants, male servants or wardsmen. Later, from the 1850s, the terms wardsmen, head wardsman and house steward appear more frequently and sometimes porter is used to denote male attendant. Collectively, however, the term 'care givers' could be referred to as hospital servants.

It is important to contextualize the several factors which make up the relationship between the British government's rationale for colonial expansion and the subsequent establishment of a colonial health service because the two are intimately connected. British gaols, by the late eighteenth century, were overcrowded and the responsibility for addressing the problem fell to Lord Sydney, Home Secretary (1783–89) in the Pitt Government (1783–1801).[4] Consequently, in 1786 the decision to establish the penal settlement in New South Wales was taken. Captain Arthur Phillip was appointed the commander of the First Fleet and the first governor of the colony.[5] The fleet comprised eleven ships and carried 775 prisoners, ten medical members and four companies of marines.[6] It departed from Portsmouth in early May 1787 and arrived off the coast of New South Wales around 18 January 1788. Phillip made settlement at Sydney Cove on 26 January.[7] Since one of the first undertakings of Phillip was to establish health facilities for the sick convicts, marines and the very few free settlers, it is clear that the British penal system, the convicts, the rationale for the settlement of New South Wales, the British military organization and the beginnings of colonial health are all intricately connected. The discussion of the history of care giving and the evolution of health facilities in colonial Australia is compartmentalized under the following headings: purpose, chronology, recent historiography, the medical staff of the first fleet, the first hospital, the extension of health facilities, the organization of the care attendants, the Sydney hospital, the Bigge report and the introduction of female nursing.

The purpose of this chapter is twofold. First, I shall examine trends connected with health care in the period under discussion as well as some associated historiographical issues. These issues are bound up with the image of the convict, health care, British social attitudes, the invisibility and the status of woman in nineteenth-century society. The second aim is to make visible the role of the male and female care givers within the context of how health care was structured and delivered. The two central themes concern the transition from the untrained attendant, both male and female, to the trained practitioner and the image of women in colonial society. This latter theme is especially important in the context of the introduction of female nursing because it was through the creation of work seen worthy for women that Florence Nightingale's reforms of the late nineteenth century provided opportunities for the betterment of a hitherto poorly regarded section of the community.

To illuminate these themes, attention is directed towards evidence which indicates how the dominance of the untrained male attendant was sustained and how the shift in emphasis from male care giver to that of the skilled female practitioner was effected. At the outset it is important to note that a serious omission in the historical record concerns the lack of narratives or letters written by the convicts themselves. This lack of testimony about early colonial social history is particularly relevant for the case of nursing. Nevertheless, from the extant sources a tentative portrayal of health care facilities, the convicts and the early care givers can be drawn. Hence the two central themes, the transition from that of unskilled attendant to that of trained practitioner and the image of women in colonial society, are considered in terms of the evolution of health care from its inception to the time of the introduction of female nursing in 1868. Both purposes are addressed through examination of the emergence of the Sydney hospital in our period.

The evolution of health care in New South Wales may be summarized as follows. Health services were mainly provided by the general hospital at Sydney which was established in 1788 and went through various metamorphoses during the years 1788–96, 1796–1816, 1816–45 and 1845–1900. As exploration opened up the colony similar institutions were established between 1788 and the mid-1830s; until the 1850s all these were subject to British military authority. The other institutions were at Parramatta (1790), and intended for general admissions. While in 1804, again at Parramatta, a factory for the colony's female workers was built and it also served as a haven for sick and poor women. In the countryside care facilities were established at Windsor (1812), Bathurst (1824), Liverpool (1828) and Goulburn (1834). The provisioning of supplies, equipment, the assignment of the care-giving staff, and who had access to the hospitals, came under military jurisdiction for the next fifty years or so.

The hospitals, intended for the convicts and the soldiers, provided medical assistance to any free person until the late 1820s when changes to the administration of health in the colony were introduced. Such changes particularly followed the Bigge report of 1823 which had been set up in 1819 to investigate the affairs of the colony during Macquarie's governorship (1810–21). Lachlan Macquarie was appointed in May 1809 as Governor of New South Wales and took up his appointment in the following year. The appointment came following a period of illegitimate government in the new colony and Macquarie's governorship was characterized by a twofold policy. First, that the essential purpose of the settlement was to improve the morals of the convicts and generally to reform the population. Second, he was enthusiastic about restoring order, encouraging peace and providing the colonists with a sense of fair treatment. In order to satisfy this policy Macquarie gave away large grants of land to the free settlers and to the emancipated convicts. Also, he spent a considerable amount of money on public works including the building of the Sydney Hospital (the 'rum hospital') believing that the convicts would be kept out of mischief by the 'moralizing effect' of employment. By the same token the free population would welcome the industry and enjoy a sense of public achievement. But Macquarie's expenditure alarmed the home authorities who subsequently, in 1819, despatched J.T. Bigge to investigate the expenditure involved and to compare the costs with other systems of punishment. Thus the period from the late 1820s until the establishment of self-government in 1851 witnessed significant changes: the gradual withdrawal of financial support for the free hospitals by the British government, the emergence of benevolent institutions, the introduction of a subscriber system and the cessation of transportation (1840).[8]

Dickey discusses colonial health and its administration in two main periods.[9] The administration by the military authorities until the late 1840s and thereafter by public charitable organizations. Conveniently, care giving and health administration are discussed here in the broad categories indicated by Dickey. The convict/ military era 1788 to the 1840s and the period between then and 1868. The central feature of colonial care-giving practice which unites the two periods is that health care delivery was primarily in the hands of men. However, changes to this situation came about in 1868 when Lucy Osburn, a *protégé* of Florence Nightingale was appointed as Lady Superintendent to the Sydney hospital. It was Osburn's responsibility to provide training in the basic skills of caring practice for the female attendants of the institution and to commence the introduction of what has become known as female nursing.

RECENT HISTORIOGRAPHY: THE CONVICT IMAGE

An examination of the historiography of the convict in early colonial Australia is important for several reasons. First, it challenges some of the myths that have come to be associated with the image of the convict, showing these to be spurious. Second, such an examination reveals the important reasons for the dominance of the male labourer in the literature and correspondingly helps to explain the reasons for the invisibility of the female domestic employee or 'nurse' for the same period. Thus recent studies offer explanation for why both the male and female care givers are difficult to perceive in the record. However, the essential reason for this is because of the small numbers involved. Finally, the analysis of the issues provides a context for the evolution of health care and sharpens the focus on the significance of Osburn's contribution.

The Australian historian Shaw cautioned as early as 1966 about accepting too readily the denigrated image of the convict: 'Overall most of the convicts were not the "atrocious villains" so often spoken of, though some of them were.'[10] On balance, the sources acknowledge that theft and alcohol were a problem for all convicts. But the severity of the image that reflects the convict person as a hardened criminal, a deviant and a sick malingerer and, in particular, depicts the female convict as a nuisance, a drain on society and an immoral creature is considered unwarranted.

First, the image of the convict as a lazy ne'er-do-well who was frequently sick: Nichol argues that the convict appears as a malingerer only because of the lack of control he/she had over the harsh and brutal working conditions. Nichol concludes that malingering was an effective mechanism for the withdrawal of labour and because of the costs to the master or government it also served as a form of 'compensatory retribution'.[11]

Convict workers

In Nicholas's *Convict Workers*, explanations may be derived from the extensive research offered as to why the male care givers are largely invisible in the convict record. This recent research presents data based on the study of 19,711 convicts in terms of the statistical evidence on occupational skills, educational background and physical fitness. For instance, Nicholas and Shergold show that convict occupations and employment are biased towards urban skills and construction technology and less towards rural skills.[12] They also explain how convict labour was organized and I indicate below how this has relevance for the way in which the care givers were assigned to the military organized health institutions.[13] Skilled convict tradesmen, sailors, shoemakers, carpenters, wheelwrights and blacksmiths were organized into workshop factories, while workers engaged in building, land clearing, road building, ploughing and thrashing were organized into gangs. The authors conclude, that, in general, assignment, supervision and incentives (additional rations) were features that the British authorities employed to structure the labour force.

We can glean a little from the studies in Nicholas's work about those men whose occupations may have fallen into the category of care attendants, if we consider male servants or domestics in this way. And in the light of Molesworth's comments in the 1838 *Report on Transportation* this is not an unreasonable consideration.[14] From the available evidence provided by Nicholas and Shergold it is possible to draw some inferences about the dominance of the male care giver and about the degree of visibility in the record of both male and female care attendants. The two main occupational groups which are to be placed near the bottom of the skill and economic pyramid are the military rank and file and domestic servants.[15] The invisibility of the male attendants in the latter record may well be connected with the small numbers involved. Out of the 19,711 convicts studied in Nicholas's work for the years 1817–40 there are 580 male convicts classified as domestic servants.[16] Based on these small numbers it is readily apparent why the male attendants are virtually imperceptible in the care-giving record. Many of these would have found employment in private assignment, leaving a still smaller number in care-giving institutions of which there were also few.

Despite the small numbers of males in the domestic servant category there are two essential reasons why their dominance in care giving and domestic work was assured for most of the nineteenth century. This state of affairs, in turn, ensured the invisibility of the female care attendant. First, as Meredith confirms, the sex-ratio was heavily biased towards males in our period, thus the virtual absence of the female care giver in the record.[17] Second, the 1838 Molesworth *Report on Transportation* reveals how women were frequently denied domestic employment because convict male servants were preferred.[18] This was the case because the poor woman in British colonial society was regarded as an outcast, being considered either a whore, a drunk, or a nuisance. The preference for male care attendants continued into the last quarter of the nineteenth century and this is especially attested to by the resistance to Osburn's efforts to introduce women as the predominant labour in care-giving practice at the Sydney Infirmary.[19]

The whore image and the female convict worker

Deborah Oxley in her study *Female Convicts* provides several reasons as to why the female convict worker has not been subsumed in the statistical analysis of the worker indicated in the broad title of Nicholas's *Convict Workers*.[20] She contends that the female convicts require distinct treatment because if they had been subsumed in the wider title, their attributes would have been obscured. Hence a separate study is warranted in order to illuminate the value of these early women. Second, another reason for dividing female from male convicts in a separate study is a matter of academic convenience. The reason is because such a division has already been made by historians and contemporaries of the convicts who condemned the male convicts for their crimes but the female convicts for their sex. Thus to counter the popular conception that convict women were a promiscuous group, Oxley examined the indents of 2,210 female convicts who arrived between 1825 and 1840. And she successfully demonstrates that the crime of 96.2 per cent of 2,191 women was petty theft (mostly clothes and cloth) and not prostitution.[21] Furthermore, the classification of the labour of 2,108 women is divided by Oxley into some thirty-seven occupations. The top two fell within the domestic servant category, 444 fell in the general servant category, 389 in the housemaid classification and the fifth and tenth occupations were classified as nursemaid and nurse, the former accounting for 189 women and the latter for only forty-two. This again demonstrates and confirms the small number of women in care giving and hence their invisibility in the record. Oxley concludes that 71.2 per cent of the females were semi-skilled and suggests, therefore, that such a result is hardly consistent with the whore image.[22]

Oxley also comments on another phenomenon which reinforces the invisibility of the female care giver in the record.[23] A characteristic feature of labour demand in the first half of the nineteenth century was the lack of demand for female labour. This lack of demand for female workers clearly reinforces the dominance of the male worker in all spheres and is bound up with the patriarchal mores of the day. The employment of women was limited, since they were regarded as unsuitable because of their alleged immoral character by the paternalistic forces of power; hence, again ensuring the dominance of the male labourer. Examples of paternalism and chauvinism abound in the sources. For instance, governor Hunter (1795–1800) stated in 1796 that he did not want any more female convicts to be transported because there was no employment for them and that they were worse characters than the men.[24] And governor Macquarie (1810–21) considered the purpose of the female factory at Parramatta as an abode for 'keeping those depraved Females at Work within the Walls'.[25] The situation was no different several decades later. In the late 1830s Molesworth stated that:

> Many respectable settlers are, however, unwilling to receive convict women, as assigned servants, when they can possibly

dispense with the services of females; and in many instances convict men-servants are preferred.[26]

However, some women were employed as companions and care givers to families. This is attested to by Peter Murdock's approach, in the 1830s, to the female factory when he intended to obtain a female servant because his wife was in 'delicate health'.[27] Gothard's analysis of single female migration to Australia demonstrates that the paternalistic attitude of the colonial government towards the female remained unchanged during the latter half of the nineteenth century:

> All colonial government female assistance schemes from the 1850's attempted to impose rigid controls over the behaviour of single female immigrants.[28]

Robinson, like Oxley, argues the case for a more positive image of the woman of last century in an attempt to counteract the influence of past paternalism and the largely patriarchically created whore image.[29] Robinson reveals that the convicted women were made of strong substance and contributed in no small manner to the establishment and growth of the colony. Robinson explains the structure of British society in the late eighteenth and for most of the nineteenth century and demonstrates how paternalism was contained within it:

> There were, in effect, two distinct societies within the normal social hierarchical structure of Britain: a society of the rich and a society of the poor – the one respectable, the other needing guidance, inducement, even threats of punishment to maintain respectability.... Once convicted of an offence, whether misdemeanour or felony, once punished by the law, the criminal man or woman was forever, a 'proven bad character' and conviction and punishment simply added confirmation to the assumptions and expectations of respectable society.[30]

Consequently, it is not surprising to find that the central thrust of the Molesworth Committee of 1837–40, set up to investigate the effects of the punishment of transportation, focuses upon the moral character of the convicts and the moral welfare of the colony.[31] Women also receive strong condemnation. Again, Peter Murdock's testimony of 1838 illustrates contemporary views on the system of punishment of the female servants:

I think to reform the unfortunate females themselves is impossible; I think they contaminated all around them; and that they were the most complete nuisance that we had in the colony.[32]

Sturma's study of the image of the fallen convict woman between 1788 and 1852 strengthens the case of contemporary society's preoccupation with the moral behaviour of women.[33] Sturma cautions that, out of the 24,000 women who were sent to the colony in that period (one-sixth of the convict population), we should be careful to consider that these were not all prostitutes but rather that the majority were ordinary working-class women possessing immediate and useful skills as domestic servants.[34] By explaining that contemporary society showed only an interest in the female convicts' moral character and less in the crime that they were condemned for, Sturma exposes the fact that the whore image arose 'from the discrepancy between working class behaviour, on the one hand, and middle-upper class expectations, on the other'.[35]

Salt encapsulates succinctly most of the foregoing when she explains the economic and social plight of the single female convict in terms of the biased sex-ratio and disdainful attitude of society:

Limited economic potential for the socially unprotected woman caused the epithet, immoral, to be generally applied to much female convict behaviour. The issue was further complicated by the numerical imbalance of the sexes. The population figures from 1821 to 1841 show a ratio of 33–50 females to 100 males. For convicts, however, the period 1787 to 1840 shows a disparity of seventeen females for every 100 males transported.[36]

The emphasis of British society on the moral state of its poorer members is an attitude which can also be identified with the medical profession. The attitude is exemplified in an 1850 article of the *Lancet*. The surgeon-superintendents, later employed on the emigrant ships in the period following the 1840s, considered it part of their duty to care for the moral character of the voyagers:

We scarcely know of a more reasonable position than that of a surgeon charged with the health, dietary, and to a certain extent, with the moral condition, of a large number of persons, of different characters and sexes.[37]

The *raison d'être* for the establishment of the colony and the essential character of the social and cultural values that the British authorities transmitted to the new settlement have been noted. These values pervade the illustrations presented and they exerted a major impact upon the division of labour which characterized care-giving practice in Australia for eighty years. The remainder of this discussion focuses on the developments regarding health care and services from 1788 and concludes with the significance of Nightingale's reforms to colonial care giving and the image of women and reforms achieved through the agency of Lucy Osburn.

MEDICAL STAFF OF THE FIRST FLEET

The initial developments regarding health care and services can be attributed to the medical members of the first fleet and the convict care givers who came out with them. Dan gives biographical detail about the ten medical members of the first fleet and notes that three of the surgeons, the Surgeon-General White, George Worgan and Bowes-Smyth are the only medical members who have had their accounts of the voyage and their experience in the first years of the new settlement published.[38] Among the more notable convicts involved in medical work from the beginning is John Irving. However, in Bowes-Smyth's journal there is mention made of a female convict, who, I suggest, may be considered the first female to be identified as a care giver in the colony.

Before departing from England in the May of 1787 on board the *Lady Penrhyn*, Bowes-Smyth, surgeon to the ships' company, listed the names of the 109 female convicts on board with their crime, age and trade attached.[39] Many of them, predictably, are described by the occupation 'domestic', but one, an Ann Smith, a 30-year-old is ascribed the title of 'nurse'. Most likely the same Smith is referred to again, approximately one year later, in the capacity of a nurse. Smith is referred to in the June 1788 diary accounts of Captain David Collins, Judge Advocate to the colony and Captain John Hunter of the *Sirius*. Smith is portrayed in the context of helping the inebriated Phebe Flarty into bed:

> On Wednesday the 4th June, Phebe Flarty was very much in liquor and had to be put to bed by Ann Smith.[40]

THE FIRST HOSPITAL AND THE FIRST CARE GIVERS

The scattered references to health matters in the diaries of the first fleeters concern illness, the medical-cum-caring facilities available and oblique as well as some direct mention of the care attendants.[41] The health of the first fleeters is generally considered to have been fair but upon disembarkation there was an outbreak of scurvy and dysentery and within three months the hospital tents which had been erected catered for over 200 patients. It soon became apparent that with so many being ill, a hospital structure was required and the first hospital building in the colony, erected some time in 1788, was a wooden one:

> eight-four feet by twenty-three, was put in hand, to be divided into a dispensary, (all the hospital-stores being at that time under tents) a ward for the troops, and another for the convicts.[42]

Nichol stresses how critical the need for hospital accommodation became when the second fleet arrived in January 1790.[43] On disembarkation, 124 deaths occurred, with another 486 scurvy-ridden survivors being admitted to the hospital. These admissions were achieved by pitching another 100 tents. The Reverend Johnson, chaplain to the new colony, provides an account which depicts the horrendous misery of these sick and, at the same time, gives us an oblique glimpse of the care givers:

> In each of these tents there were about four sick people; here they lay in a most deplorable situation. At first they had nothing to lay upon but the damp ground, many scarcely a rag to cover them. Grass was got for them to lay upon, and a blanket given amongst four of them ... many were not able to turn, or even stir themselves and in this situation were covered over almost with their own nastiness, their heads, bodies, clothes, blanket, all full of filth and lice.[44]

And each morning for a week, it was observed:

> the attendants of the sick passing frequently backwards and forwards from the hospital to the burying ground with the miserable victims of the night.[45]

THE EXTENSION OF HEALTH FACILITIES

The first hospital to be established outside of Sydney Cove was in 1790 at Rosehill, which later became known as Parramatta.[46] This hospital had been erected under the supervision of the surgeon Thomas Arndell and he received further medical assistance in 1791 when the convict physician, John Irving was assigned to the new settlement.[47] The lack of cleanliness of the health facility and the lack of attention to the patients by the care attendants is well attested. For instance, in the November 1790 report of Captain Tench, the institution is described as, 'a most wretched hospital, totally destitute of every conveniency'.[48] In 1791, Tench reported that the hospital had become 'two long sheds, built in the form of a tent' and said to have a thatched roof and a bed capacity of 200. By 1792 the sheds had become a brick building containing two wards. Salt has recorded that by 1818 these wards, each intended to accommodate fifty patients, in fact, contained ninety-five at a minimum.[49] We do not know the number of attendants but it was most likely to be insufficient and they appear to have provided inadequate care because corpses remained for days in the hospital hallway. As Nichol comments that since the convict and the rank and file soldier could not look for much in their daily lives it is not surprising that they exhibited an indifference to the wretchedness surrounding them.[50] As the colony's population grew and expansion into the outlying areas occurred, more military hospitals were built to accommodate the changes. The appearance of these hospitals spans the years from 1790 through to the mid-1830s. The first of their kind, as noted above, was at Parramatta (1790) and intended for general admissions. Later at Parramatta another institution was established in 1804 to accommodate the female convict population. The history behind the establishment of the female factory is thoroughly treated by Salt in *These Outcast Women*, however, further comment is given below. In the countryside military hospitals were built at Windsor (1812), at Bathurst (1824), at Liverpool (1828) and at Goulburn (1834).

THE ORGANIZATION OF THE CARE ATTENDANTS

The allocation of the care attendants to these military institutions, in the first instance, was the responsibility of the superintendent of convicts and, in the second, that of the surgeon-general.[51] It was the common practice that the superintendent inspected the prisoners on disembarkation and assigned prisoners to the task that best suited their past work experience.[52] Thus the superintendent assigned the convict either to the workshop or to the work 'gang' and allocated overseers from among the convicts to supervise. By analogy it is reasonable to infer that those who fell within the category of care attendants and overseers of the care attendants were assigned through a similar process. Thus it may be inferred that the superintendent of convicts in conjunction with the surgeon-general inspected the convicts on arrival and assigned them accordingly. Hence, the physician convict John Irving was assigned an assistant medical role in the hospital at Sydney Cove in the early days of 1788 and he was later transferred, with the same role, to the hospital at Parramatta in 1791.[53] At the same time, the nurse Ann Smith appears to have been assigned to the caring role of the female patients. This conclusion about the allocation of the care worker is further supported by the fact that in the 1838 Molesworth *Report on Transportation* there is an example given of one Peter Montgomery, 'a convict employed as overseer at the Liverpool hospital'.[54] However, the care givers are shadowy figures and the obscurity of processes involved in allocating them to work roles and places reinforces the fact that few were involved and the silence of the sources in these matters reflects the value placed on their work.

However, clues about the functioning and the organization of the first hospital at Sydney Cove are reflected in an intriguing incident from 1788. It involves the medical staff, some convict attendants and some convicts in-charge of hospital supplies.[55] On 3 July, a convict, Thomas Chadwick reported to surgeon-general White that the patients' wine needed replenishing and the surgeon ordered the bottles to be filled. About midnight White was awakened by the noise of vomiting and found, with the medical assistants Balmain and Arndell, that Chadwick, as well as two other convicts connected with the hospital staff, Joshua Peck and John Small, were in states of 'beastly drunkenness'. White also inspected the hospital servants and found them all asleep in their bed.

What can be said about the quality of care and the division of labour in the early period (1788–1820s) of the existence of the caring facilities? Dingwall, Rafferty and Webster have pointed to

the difficulties in identifying care-giving practices as nursing and
non-nursing in the days before 'modern' nursing began to be
codified.[56] However, it is possible to make some remarks about
the duties of the attendants in this period and in the light of the
evidence provided above, it must also be concluded that the
attendants provided limited care. It appears that the male attendants were concerned with the supervision of male patients, the
diet and the burial of patients. Duties of a similar kind can most
likely be inferred for the female attendants in respect to looking
after the female patients. In addition to these duties the attendants gave little, if any, attention to the patients' hygiene, toileting
and bathing. Dressings, poultices and medicines were usually
undertaken by the medical members. Later, in the 1820s and after,
the medical member or his assistant dispensed the medicines
to the attendants to give the patients.[57] In regard to the division
of labour, it has been established that there were more men than
women in the colony and this is a factor to consider when concluding that health care practices were largely in the hands of
men. The other crucial element is that the sociocultural mores
of the day led the authorities to consider poor women as unsuitable to employ in any capacity.

The one institution in the colony which came to have predominantly female staff under the charge of a matron was the female
factory at Parramatta established in 1804 and rebuilt in 1818. Salt
explains that it was built to provide refuge for unmarried women
and was seen as a way of employing women for some useful
economic purpose.[58] Originally, a gaol erected in the time of
governor King (1800–06), the upper floor was utilized as a place
of punishment for women convicts. The rest of the building was
used to some extent either as an asylum, or for those in need of
confinement, or for those who were ill or again, as a house
of industry, particularly for the manufacture of woollen goods.
By 1817 it was clear that the accommodation was inadequate
because the factory could only house sixty of the 200 women it
employed. Thus governor Macquarie, in 1818, arranged for the
construction of a new female factory which was completed in
1821. The new building could house 300 women and was built on
a four-acre site opposite the old gaol.[59]

Initially, the superintendents who had sole management of the
factory were men and the first person in charge when the factory
was operating above the gaol was a convict.[60] However, the col-

onial authorities augmented the administration of the female factory in April 1824 by the appointment of a matron, Elizabeth
Fulloon, and she remained until 1827. In 1827, Ann Gordon took
over the role until 1836. Salt has recorded that by this time the
factory's administration comprised assistant matrons who were
frequently soldiers' wives, a storekeeper-superintendent, a port-
ress, monitress and a constable gatekeeper.[61] In addition to these
staff there was a board of management and a ladies' committee.
During Mrs Gordon's period and by 1828 there were 490 convicts
and five women employed to care for them.[62] In regard to the
housekeeping and moral supervisory functions of the matron it
is to be noted that it is through this very role that Nightingale
effected the transition of the supervision of labour power from
the male administrator to the female superintendent. This transition in roles and power is especially exemplified in 1868 by the
appointment of Osburn, as the lady superintendent to the Sydney
infirmary.

Thus the female factory, originally intended as a penitentiary
and a workshop, soon served as a labour bureau for those seeking
domestic servants and a place for sick women or those in confinement.[63] The quality of the medical care was dependent on the
surgeon's personal whim to make a visit.[64] I hesitate to infer
anything about the quality of care that the occupants may have
given one another in view of the riotous reputation of the factory
and the prevalence of disease and unhygienic conditions.[65] Further
changes to the staffing arrangements can be detected in 1836
when a Mr and Mrs Bell were appointed as keeper and matron
at a time when it was considered as respectable for a married
couple to be in charge. And associated with these changes is the
fact that for the first time, in 1837, a salaried midwife, Mary
Mumford, was also employed.[66]

The character of the institution altered again in the late 1840s.
Transportation ceased in 1840 and as a result, the assignment of
female labour to outside services also stopped. By this time the
institution was caring for 590 women and 136 children. What had
begun as a gaol-cum-workhouse became a lying-in hospital and
nursery. Again changes to the administration followed in 1848
when a Mr and Mrs Edwin Statham were employed as the keeper
and matron. The composition of the patients also altered. It now
became an asylum for the poor and the infirm, male and female,
and it also admitted those categorized as insane. By the 1850s

the staff consisted of twenty-one persons, a dispenser, and a head nurse and head wardsman were among these.

THE SYDNEY HOSPITAL 1816–45

By the first decade of the nineteenth century the wooden hospital at Sydney Cove no longer served the needs of the increasing population and with the arrival of governor Macquarie in 1810 a new and substantial hospital of eight wards was begun. This became known as the famous 'rum hospital'. It opened its doors in 1816 and the composition of the staff, the organization of care and the quality of care are features which show up quite clearly in the record from now on.[67] The convict care attendants comprised an overseer, an attendant clerk, a gatekeeper, a matron, and a number of male and female care givers.[68]

Included in the daily activities of the hospital was the visit of the surgeon in the mornings to attend the patients; he was accompanied by the overseer, a clerk and a care attendant.[69] Prescriptions were ordered and the clerk recorded these. Dressings were attended to by the medical assistant or medical dresser. After the surgeon had completed his round he went to the stores and issued what was required and medicines were dispensed by the medical assistant and passed to the care givers to administer. It may be inferred from Watson's (1911) account that the nursing responsibilities, bathing, feeding, toileting and scrubbing and cleaning were often not done. The patients were mustered every evening and, with no attendants, were locked in the wards between 9 p.m. and 6 a.m. Cleanliness was notable by its absence given that the bed was changed only weekly and then usually by the patients themselves. Thus it is of little surprise to find that vermin inhabited the beds.

Toileting was not a high priority since the toilets were outside and inaccessible to patients at night. And during the day those patients who were very sick crawled to the facilities on their hands and knees.[70] There was no mortuary and one of the kitchens was utilized for the purpose while the other kitchen, twelve yards away from the patients, was occupied by the overseer and a male attendant.[71] In the absence of the kitchens, food was cooked in the wards by the patients themselves. Nichol, citing evidence given to the Bigge inquiry (discussed below), by some of those who worked in the institution confirms the poor care-giving practices.[72] The female nurses, chiefly selected from the female factory at Parramatta, were frequently inebriated and it was not unknown for the attendants to pilfer from the patients.[73] Further changes in the Sydney Hospital occurred between 1819 and 1927 when Bowman became the principal surgeon and then in 1827, Inspector of Colonial Hospitals.[74] At this time there was an increase in the number of care attendants and changes to the daily routine. In addition to the increase of male and female care givers, the staff now consisted of an overseer, an assistant clerk, two cooks, two gatekeepers (one for the outside gate and one for the female ward), and a dispenser. Better dietary scales were introduced, linen was not washed in the wards and clean linen was issued as required, wards were cleaned every morning between 6 a.m. and 8 a.m., windows were left open at night to allow for better ventilation, commodes were provided in the vestibules and order was maintained at night because nurses and wardsmen now slept in the wards. However, in the light of the conditions which prevailed at this institution in the 1860s and which compelled Sir Henry Parks to seek the assistance of Nightingale to overcome the absence of cleanliness, sanitation and compassion, it must be concluded that the efforts of Bowman were short-lived.

THE BIGGE REPORT, 1823

Other relevant changes in the evolution of health care in New South Wales took place between 1810 and the 1850s, that is from the beginning of Macquarie's governorship through until the time of self-government. The Bigge Report, the beginnings of private health organizations and the events leading up to the metamorphosis of the Sydney rum hospital into the Sydney Infirmary and Dispensary in 1845, are the most salient. It was to this latter institution that Osburn introduced female nursing. Prior to the arrival of Macquarie and up to about the late 1830s medical assistance and hospital facilities were free to settlers, soldiers and convicts – the so called 'open door' policy. However, during the time of Macquarie and after, the colonists came to realize that the British government would not continue to financially support this policy of free access to health facilities. Indeed, the colonists' fears were confirmed when Bigge's report of 1823 found fault with the government's open door policy and thus the relevance of this inquiry is that it brought alterations to the structure of health care in colonial Australia. As noted above, Bigge had been sent out in 1819 to New South Wales to investigate Macquarie's well-intentioned but extravagant public works and public health initiatives and he concluded that the public purse could no longer meet the health demands of the people of New South Wales. Thus in view of the impending economic changes occurring during Macquarie's time, charitable institutions other than the Sydney Hospital came into existence. For example, in 1818, the Benevolent Society of New South Wales was established and in 1826, the Sydney Dispensary was in operation (largely servicing outpatients). Following the Bigge Report and by the 1830s, private benevolence had become a permanent feature of colonial society. Changes came about then as can be detected in the restraining of the public purse, the emergence of private benevolent organizations, and by the mid-nineteenth century, the establishment of the subscriber system. Nichol connects the tightening up of the admission criteria for the non-convict population to a deterioration in Sydney's public health because most of the population were paupers.[75] However, the benevolent movement continued into the 1840s with the creation of the Sydney Infirmary in 1845. This was an amalgamation of the Sydney Hospital and the Dispensary and thereafter was known as the Sydney Infirmary and Dispensary.

LUCY OSBURN AND THE SYDNEY INFIRMARY AND DISPENSARY

Between the mid-1850s and the arrival in 1868 of Lucy Osburn, the Sydney Infirmary was managed by a board of directors elected annually by the subscribers. During this time the wardsmen and the female care givers who tallied around twenty-three male and five female were largely drawn from among the reformed convict population, since transportation had ceased in 1840. The administration suffered rivalries between board members and staff and, in general, mismanagement prevailed. In 1867 a male superintendent was appointed to take charge of all the servants and the daily management of the institution.[76] However, the chaotic state of affairs at the hospital were notorious and this led Sir Henry Parkes, the famous politician of New South Wales, to write in the July of 1866 to Florence Nightingale with a request to introduce trained nursing into the Sydney Infirmary. He characterized the conditions at the Infirmary:

> Among the subjects which engaged my attention on my
> entrance into public life was the care and treatment of the sick
> and insane in the Government asylums. There was at that time
> but one general hospital in the city of Sydney; and that was
> under a very unsatisfactory system of management .... This
> circumstance led me to a personal inspection of the wards and
> the condition of the inmates, and to enquiries as to the staff
> of attendants and the general treatment of the patients. As the
> result of my investigation, I sent a communication to Miss
> Nightingale requesting her services in engaging a staff of
> trained nurses for the colony.[77]

Nightingale responded in October 1866. Arrangements were
made for the departure of Lucy Osburn and five others for New
South Wales and they arrived in the March of 1868. Russell draws
attention to the horrendous conditions which confronted Osburn.
The presence of vermin, the lack of water, the lack of sanitation
and the general absence of compassion were characteristic of the
institution. Indeed, Russell reinforces the image of the careless
male and female attendants when she notes that the patients
were allowed to lie in unmade beds unwashed for weeks and it
was apparently put forward by the attendants that: 'the doctor
said they were not to be disturbed.'[78]

The management problems which confronted Osburn relate
directly to the hospital's preference for male care givers. It was
understood by Osburn that she was to be Superintendent and
Chief Female Officer of the Sydney Infirmary, in charge of all
the female labour. This was not understood by the hospital
authorities. What essentially lay behind the thrust of Nightingale's
intention and Osburn too, was to introduce what has come to
be known as female nursing. Osburn and her nurses were to be
responsible for the training of the other female attendants in the
practice of good nursing care. However, neither the manager nor
the medical authorities saw any merit in having females do the
nursing at all.[79]

Russell clarifies the change in nursing from that of a predominantly male-centred care-giving attendance to that of female practice. One of the distinctive characteristics of Nightingale's system
was to bring about a different role for the matron.[80] Prior to

Nightingale's time the matron had little influence over the actual caring of the sick. The role was chiefly a domestic one of house-keeping, managing the stores, the linen supply, the kitchen oper-ations, the laundry, the sewing and the cleaning. In a letter of 1867, Nightingale makes it clear how she envisaged the change in roles between the male administrator and the female care giver:

> to take all power over the Nursing out of the hands of man, and put it into the hands of one female trained head and make her responsible for everything (regarding the internal management and discipline) being carried out.[81]

Consequently, once Nightingale's system effected the change in the role of the matron it was a small step to the introduction of female nursing generally and the reduction in the numbers and dominance of the male care attendants.

CONCLUSION

In broad terms there are two fundamental contributions of Night-ingale which revolutionized the image of the care giver and care-giving practice by the late nineteenth century. First, Nightingale brought to the profession of nursing an elevated status to women as care givers. She was able to do this through bringing about an altered perception of several of British society's attitudes and values. The attitudes held by the authorities towards the poor were, as we have seen, that they considered them depraved and unworthy in general, and that women of a particular social class were wretched and promiscuous. Nightingale altered the view of those who considered themselves the agents of moral welfare and by so doing she opened up opportunities for the not-so-privileged class of woman to gain a worthwhile and respectable livelihood. In view of the strong convictions of British society that the less privileged class of women were not preferred as care givers, it is remarkable that one person could have such influence in bringing about change. Baly's citation of Nightingale's favourite saying: 'you cannot be a good nurse without being a good woman' must be located in the context of the late nineteenth-century changes.[82] It is appropriate to mention that the received view of the unre-formed care giver as one lacking compassion and kindliness has to be considered with a certain degree of scepticism given that the reforming faction was motivated to paint a bleak picture of the care-giving practices of the past. Nightingale's other outstanding contribution is that she wrote down the regulations by which the training of women in the practice of nursing could take place. Nightingale's 1858 *Notes on Nursing What it is and What it is Not* is famous. However, Brodsky makes relevant comment about another text of Nightingale's, *The Method of Improving Nursing Service of Hospitals*, and a copy of this, inscribed by the doyen herself, was given to Osburn and today it is held at the Sydney Hospital.[83] Thus Nightingale and education altered the status and the image of women in nursing. It is these factors which lay behind the transformation of care-giving practices in New South Wales and the introduction of female nursing by Lucy Osburn into colonial Australia in 1868.

NOTES

1 B. Schultz, *A Tapestry of Service, The Evolution of Nursing in Australia 1788–1900*, Melbourne, Churchill Livingstone, vol. 1, 1991.

2 A. Cushing, ' "Bartz Schultz, Tapestry of Service, Evolution of Nursing In Australia 1788–1900, Vol 1"', *Colnursa*, 1992, vol. 11, p. 5.

3 A. Cushing, *A Contextual Perspective to Female Nursing in Victoria, 1850–1914*, Victoria, Deakin University Press, 1993, p. 10.

4 J. Moore, *The First Fleet Marines, 1786–1792*, St Lucia, University of Queensland Press, Queensland, 1987, pp. 18–24.

5 The military governors of New South Wales in chronological order are:
   Phillip (1788–92); Interregnum (1792–95); Hunter (1795–1800); King (1800–06); Bligh (1806–09); Interregnum (1809–10); Macquarie (1810–21); Brisbane (1821–25); Darling (1825–31); Bourke (1831–38); Gipps (1838–46) and Fitzroy (1846–55).

6 Figures vary in the sources. For example, N. Dan, in J. Pearn and C. O'Carrigan (eds), *Australia's Quest for Colonial Health*, Brisbane, Department of Child Health, Royal Children's Hospital, Brisbane, 1983, p. 4 give 775, W. Nichol, 'Brothels, Slaughter Houses and Prisons', *Push from the Bush*, 1986, vol. 22, p. 7 gives 759.

7 J. Cobley, *Sydney Cove*, London, Hodder & Stoughton, 1962, p. 5 for relevant comment about the chronology associated with Phillip's exploration of Botany Bay and Port Jackson in January 1788.

8 During the governorships of Gipps (1838–46) and Fitzroy (1846–55) changes to the administration of the colony came about. First in 1842 the Constitutional Act was passed creating a Legislative Council and in 1851 the Elective Act, creating two houses and self-government.

9 B. Dickey, 'Health and the State in Australia, 1788–1977', *Journal of Australian Studies*, 1977, vol. 1, pp. 50–63.

10 A.G.L. Shaw, *Convicts and the Colonies*, Melbourne, Melbourne University Press, 1981, p. 164.
11 W. Nichol, ' "Malingering" and Convict Protest', *Labour History*, 1984, vol. 47, Nov., pp. 18–20 and 27.
12 S. Nicholas and P. Shergold, 'Unshackling the Past', in S. Nicholas (ed) *Convict Workers: Reinterpreting Australia's Past*, Cambridge, Cambridge University Press, 1988, p. 11.
13 Ibid.
14 Sir William Molesworth, *Report from Select Committee of the House of Commons on Transportation and Notes by Sir William Molesworth, Henry Hooper*, London, p. 12.
15 Nicholas and Shergold, op. cit., p. 68.
16 Ibid.
17 D. Meredith, 'Full Circle? Contemporary Views on Transportation' in S. Nicholas, op. cit., p. 17.
18 Sir William Molesworth, op. cit., p. 12.
19 J.F. Watson, *The History of Sydney Hospital, from 1811–1911*, Sydney, University of New South Wales Press, 1964.
20 D. Oxley, 'Female Convicts' in S. Nicholas, op. cit., p. 85.
21 Ibid, p. 89.
22 Ibid, p. 92.
23 Ibid, p. 95.
24 B. Schultz, op. cit., p. 11.
25 A. Salt, *These Outcast Women*, Sydney, Hale & Iremonger, 1984, p. 99.
26 Ibid, p. 12.
27 Sir William Molesworth, PP 1837–8 XXII C669, Answer 1443, p. 118.
28 J. Gothard, in E. Richards (ed.), *Visible Immigrants: Two*, Dept of History and Centre for Immigration and Multicultural Studies, Research School of Social Sciences, Australian National University, Canberra, 1991, pp. 97–116.
29 P. Robinson, *The Women of Botany Bay*, Sydney, Macquarie Library, 1988, p. 6.
30 Ibid., p. 151.
31 Sir William Molesworth, PP. 1837–8, XXII, C669; Question 549, p. 57; Question 718, p. 69.
32 Ibid., C669 Answer 1443, p. 118.
33 M. Sturma, 'Eye of the Beholder: The Stereotype of Women Convicts, 1788–1852', *Labour History*, 1978, vol. 34, pp. 3–17.
34 Ibid., p. 3.
35 Ibid., p. 4.
36 Ibid., p. 39.
37 Anonymous author, 'Surgeons of Immigrant Ships', *Lancet*, 1850, vol. ii, p. 328.
38 N. Dan, in Pearn and O'Carrigan, op. cit., pp. 3–12.
39 P.G. Fidlon and R.J. Ryan (eds), *The Journal of Arthur Bowes-Smyth: Surgeon, Lady Penrhyn 1787–1789*, Australian Documents Library, 1979, Sydney, 39, pp. 4–8.
40 Cobley, op. cit., p. 161.

41 Dan, op. cit., pp. 1–4; Watt, op. cit., pp. 846–7; Cobley, op. cit., p. 48–9.
42 Cobley, op. cit., pp. 48–9.
43 Nichol, 1986, op. cit., pp. 8–9.
44 Ibid., p. 9.
45 Ibid.
46 Cobley, op. cit., p. 245.
47 D. Richards, 'Transported to New South Wales: Medical Convicts 1788–1850', *British Medical Journal*, 1987, vol. 295, pp. 1609–12.
48 Nichol, op. cit., p. 9.
49 Salt, op. cit., pp. 44 and 111.
50 Nichol, op. cit., p. 10.
51 C. White, *Journal of a Voyage to New South Wales*, originally published in 1790, with an Introduction by Rex Rientis and Alec H. Chisholm (eds), Sydney, Angus and Robertson, 1962, p. 135; J.F. Watson, op. cit., p. 50.
52 Sir William Molesworth, op. cit., Report from the Select Committee of the House of Commons on Transportation and notes, Henry Hooper, London, p. 9.
53 Dan, op. cit., p. 3.
54 Sir William Molesworth, op. cit., Report from the Select Committee of the House of Commons on Transportation and notes, Henry Hooper, London, p. 34.
55 Cobley, op. cit., pp. 173–4.
56 R. Dingwall, A.M. Rafferty and C. Webster, *An Introduction to the Social History of Nursing*, London, Routledge, 1988.
57 Watson, op. cit., p. 39.
58 Salt, op. cit., pp. 40–3.
59 Ibid., p. 48 and 50.
60 Ibid., p. 56–7.
61 Ibid., p. 58.
62 Schultz, op. cit., p. 12.
63 Salt, op. cit., p. 112.
64 Ibid., p. 58.
65 Ibid., pp. 94, 113–6.
66 Ibid., p. 113; Schultz, op. cit., p. 12 reveals that the suggestion that a midwife be employed was first made nine years earlier, in 1828.
67 Watson, op. cit., p. 33.
68 Ibid., p. 36.
69 Ibid., p. 39.
70 Ibid., p. 42.
71 Nichol, 1986, op. cit., p. 15.
72 Ibid., pp. 15–6.
73 Ibid., p. 16.
74 Ibid., p. 48 and W. Nichol, 'Medicine and the Labour Movement in New South Wales, 1788–1850', *Labour History*, 1985, vol. 49, pp. 18–19. This author cautions about accepting too readily Watson's account of Bowman's salubrious effect on the Sydney hospital.
75 Nichol, 1985, op. cit., p. 30.

76 Watson, op. cit., p. 121.
77 Sir Henry Parkes, *Fifty Years in the Making of Australian History*, Vol I, Books for Libraries Press, reprinted 1971, Freeport, New York, p. 207.
78 L. Russell, 'Training of Nurses at the Lucy Osburn School of Nursing', *Educational Inquiry*, 1979, vol. 2, pp. 35–54.
79 M. Anderson, 'The Women's Movement' in M. Atkinson (ed.), *Australia: Economic and Political Studies*, Macmillan, London, 1920, p. 284; Watson, op. cit., p. 141.
80 L. Russell, *From Nightingale to Now*, W.B. Saunders, Sydney, 1990, pp. 11–13.
81 Ibid., p. 11.
82 M. Baly, *Florence Nightingale and the Nursing Legacy*, Croom Helm, Beckenham, 1986, p. 25.
83 I. Brodsky, *Sydney's Nurse Crusaders*, Sydney, Old Sydney Free Press, 1968, p. 22.

Chapter 7

Independent women: domiciliary nurses in mid-nineteenth-century Edinburgh

Barbara Mortimer

she is laying by: she goes every quarter to the Bank in Millcote. I should not wonder but she has saved enough to keep her independent if she liked to leave; but I suppose she's got used to the place; and she's not forty yet, and strong and able for anything. It is too soon for her to give up business.[1]

The possibility that one of that shadowy group of women, the early nineteenth-century domiciliary nurses, could be viewed as a successful businesswoman is perhaps surprising, but the increasingly wealthy, sophisticated and leisured middle classes of the first half of the nineteenth century generated a demand for their services. There is no dispute that such women were employed to work in private homes. However, the unreformed early nineteenth-century domiciliary nurse is the most elusive of creatures. She appeared fleetingly in diaries and novels where she assisted with critical family events including birth, death, sickness and madness. A variety of fictional nurses were created, the most renowned of whom was presented by Dickens in the person of Sarah Gamp, midwife, layer-out and sick nurse. Although this thoroughly entertaining character in *Martin Chuzzlewit* (1844) was a caricature, her distinctly seedy image in 'a very rusty black gown, rather the worse for snuff', has survived. Mid-nineteenth-century readers could place the fictional portraits into their contemporary context, but the alarming image of Dickens' unreformed nurse was so useful to the arguments of later reformers that this became the reference point they adopted. No systematic attempt has since been made to determine whether or not that image was deserved. For the twentieth-century reader the fictional image rests in the context of later propaganda which it is hard to evaluate. The real nurses – who they were and how they managed their lives – remain mysterious.

Anne Summers has suggested that a large number of the women who were returned as 'nurse, not domestic servant' in the 1861 census report for central London might have been independent practitioners working in competition with doctors for areas of general practice.[2] Certainly towards the end of the century when state registration for nurses was being canvassed, some doctors, struggling to make a living in a limited market, expressed a fear of such a challenge.[3] In another essay Summers analysed the problems experienced in the Crimea when 'lady volunteers' were expected to work alongside 'professional' hospital nurses. No precedent existed to guide their conduct. Summers cited Lady Canning who commented despairingly on the difference between the hardened institutional nurses and the much more acceptable 'private nurses' described by Summers as 'lower class women who knew their place'.[4] At least three groups of nurses can be discerned from contemporary accounts: hospital nurses, independent practitioners and 'private' domiciliary nurses. Summers commented that Sarah Gamp combined the roles of a domiciliary nurse and an independent practitioner who was called in as a consultant by her fellows. The domiciliary nurses of the first half of the century worked at a time when professional boundaries in the medical world were being redefined.[5] Undoubtedly some nurses worked as independent practitioners, the most unambiguous group being the midwives, but the little which is known to date suggests that the total picture was complex.

This chapter seeks to trace something of the lives and work of those women who defined themselves as domiciliary nurses and worked in the first half of the nineteenth century in Edinburgh. The city provides an ideal case study; it was small (168,121 or 6 per cent of the Scottish population in 1861), wealthy, and a centre of medical excellence. A particularly attractive civic environment had been created since the late eighteenth century with the building of the New Town. The New Town was a planned classical city, of wide gracious streets lined by the grand houses of the rich and fashionable. Between the principal streets were lanes and mews where the more modest dwellings of those providing services for the wealthy were located. Almost one-third of the city's population was classified as 'middle class', more than in any other Scottish city, reflecting the concentration of legal, financial and educational institutions in the capital.[6] With this environment Edinburgh had developed as a significant centre of medical consultation. The medical school was very well known and a number of its doctors were national figures including perhaps the most eminent obstetrician of his day, James Young Simpson, Professor of Medicine, Midwifery and the Diseases of Children, and Physician to the Queen in Scotland. By the middle of the nineteenth century most of the fashionable doctors had homes or consulting rooms in the New Town. In the same area were the hotels and lodgings used by visitors. The census of 1861 reported that 265 or 17 per cent of the Scottish women who were returned as 'nurse not domestic servant' lived in Edinburgh.[7]

The working lives of nineteenth-century women are notoriously difficult to uncover. For the present study the Post Office directories of the city of Edinburgh 1834–71 and the enumerators' books of the census of 1861 have provided data, the value of which have been enhanced by linking the two records.[8] Both these records, like most others, were created by men in an environment which valued women's paid work lightly. A powerful assumption underpinning the creation of such records was that women should be located within a 'protected' domestic environment, which usually meant a household headed by a man. Such social constraints severely limited the options available to unsupported women who could easily find themselves insecure and economically marginalized. It was well known that the major users of the Poor Law were women and their dependent children.

In 1861, 145 women were listed as 'midwives', 'sick nurses' or 'lady's nurses' in the Edinburgh Post Office directory. This included eighty-seven in the 'professional' section. The annual Post Office directories of Edinburgh included three types of listing. Professional directory entries were listed alphabetically under selected professional descriptors; for nurses these were 'midwife' and 'sick nurse'.[9] The 'street' directory listed the city streets alphabetically with householders' names. Finally the 'general' directory listed all individuals alphabetically. An occupational descriptor could be included in the last two lists and this might differ from those in the 'professional' directory. The most common additional descriptor for nurses was 'lady's nurse'. Some nurses opted for entry in all three lists and many used all three of the major descriptors. All groups are included in this discussion.

Why should 145 women choose to be listed in the directory,

something which many chose to do over long periods of time? Mrs Elizabeth Duncan of 21 Jamaica Street was consistently recorded in the directory from the same address between 1851 and 1871, and many more examples could be cited. When seeking to estimate the significance to nurses of entry in the directories, it is clearly important to consider why they were compiled and the environment within which they were used. Morris, while acknowledging that such publications could act as a 'social register' concluded that their primary function was utilitarian or commercial. He considered that such a guide would ensure an individual's location 'in an increasingly complex world of business and commerce.'[10]

There are some features of the nursing entries which are different from any others. As a group nurses have been compared with 'the better class of domestic servants', yet domestic servants never appear in these directories. Nurses were employed intermittently, they were seen and saw themselves in a different relationship with their employers. It was noticeable in the census enumerators' books that nurses were often entered first or last in a list of servants, and in 'relation to head of household' they were frequently identified by a professional descriptor and not simply as 'servant'. Only women were included in the professional lists which seem to have been deliberately structured in that way; very small numbers of men appeared elsewhere in all the directories. Two men advertised in 1861 as 'attendant on invalid gentlemen' and 'gentleman's sick nurse' respectively. The other major female occupations in the professional directory were 'milliners and dressmakers', and 'stay and corset makers', although neither was an exclusively female occupation. These two occupations can readily be recognized as commercial enterprises and the value of an entry to customers and fellow tradesmen is easily understood. When interpreting the data it is important to recall that the service offered by nurses was seen by them as fitting into this commercial world.

The most closely related occupation listed was 'medical practitioner'. The list of 'medical practitioners' seems comprehensive but apart from indicating the practitioners who were unregistered, no professional qualifications were included. The doctors invested little effort in submitting details; they appreciated the convenience for tradesmen and their patients of ready access to an address but they were not attempting to impress or convince uncommitted patients. Since 1858 full professional information relating to all the qualified doctors had been published in the Medical Register, the existence of which nurses at this time must have been aware. Nurses might seek inclusion in the directory for convenience as did the doctors, but for nurses there might have been added value. Those with professional ambition might value inclusion in the same volume as the medical men whether they regarded themselves as competitors or partners. Directory entry for these women may have been in part a statement of their personal estimation of worth or an indication of their personal ambition. For them it may have been a serious and public indication of their occupational focus, implying some degree of competence and success. This was the closest they could get to entry in an official publication which mimicked, in part, the approach taken by the doctors. At the very least it provided an accurate record of their current address and implied some expectation of permanence.

Another issue which needs to be considered is the nature of the client group. The directory gives a very clear guide to this. An analysis of entries between 1834 and 1871 indicates that although only two descriptors were used in the professional directory ('midwife' and 'sick nurse') from the very earliest directories some nurses had described themselves as 'lady's nurse' in the 'street' and 'general' directories. The numbers of women using this latter descriptor increased steadily over time (see Table 7.1)

Table 7.1 Changes in the nurse population of Edinburgh: lady's nurse

	1834	1841	1851	1861	1871
All 'nurses'	82	103	140	145	167
Lady's nurse	3	21	65	105	142
Percentage	4	20	46	72	85

Source: Post Office directories of Edinburgh and Leith, 1834–71

These figures clearly demonstrate the increasing economic importance that care of post-natal women had for domiciliary nurses in Edinburgh. A picture of the normal work of a 'lady's nurse' emerged from the enumerators' books of the 1861 census. The majority at work on census night were caring for women within a month of child-birth. The precise nature of their work is indicated in various manuals published during the nineteenth century and aimed at nurses.[11] Some advice was offered to potential employers in such volumes as Mrs Beeton's *Household Management* (1861).[12] Nurses were expected to be resident just before the birth and for about a month afterwards. They attended to all the personal needs of the mother and infant and accepted responsibility for some domestic tasks, depending on the size of the staff. Normally only one nurse was employed who gave twenty-four-hour personal care, and took her own rest when she could. The fees paid to these nurses are unclear but Miss Nightingale in 1859 spoke of them earning 'their guinea a week'. However, pay for servants in Scotland was normally less than in England. Since each booking guaranteed an income for a month or so, this work was often preferred to sick nursing which was more unpredictable. Securing an adequate income from such an occupation would require some organizational skills and a good communication network. In addition to the client group of middle-class residents of Edinburgh the presence of a transient population of individuals visiting the city to seek medical advice is attested to by contemporary observers.[13]

Reflecting once again on the value of a directory entry in the light of the major client groups, it seems inconceivable that respectable middle-class women, some of whom had travelled to the city expressly to consult a particular doctor, would engage such a close body servant or carer as a monthly nurse simply from information contained in a directory. Indeed there is evidence to suggest the contrary. However, in a city where a significant proportion of the client group were likely to be transients a serious businesswoman would surely seek to exploit every avenue to corroborate her skills and demonstrate that she was well known.

Since the directory was likely to play only a part in the process of employing a nurse other resources must have been used. The role of doctors as intermediaries is attested to by a number of letters within the correspondence of the eminent obstetrician James Young Simpson which indicate both that society ladies travelled to Edinburgh to be attended by him and that they sought his advice in selecting a monthly nurse.[14] Simpson worked in Edinburgh from his graduation in 1832 until just before his death in 1870. In a notebook of his dating from around 1840 he logged information about nurses, some of whom were listed in the directories.[15] Doubtless networks existed of women who recommended nurses to each other but it seems to have been accepted that men also played a part in finding a nurse. John Gulland in 1848 recorded how his father and uncle searched the city for a wet nurse after his aunt died, and John Inglis recommended the monthly nurse who had cared for his wife to a male friend whose wife was pregnant.[16,17] If men had a significant role to play in this process, then the presence of the nurses in a document which was an established part of the male business world is totally logical.

In order to enhance our understanding of these domiciliary nurses the enumerators' books of the 1861 census were examined. The published census report recorded 265 women described as 'nurse, not domestic servant'.[18] Scanning the enumerators' books produced a sample of 946 individuals assigned an occupation which might be defined as 'nursing'. More than thirty different descriptors contributed to this total. Comparing the enumerators' books with the census reports indicated that the census clerks appear to have included within the group 'nurse, not domestic servant', hospital nurses working in the Royal Infirmary of Edinburgh (RIE) and all those working outside institutions described as 'lady's nurse', 'sick nurse', 'monthly nurse' and 'professed or professional nurse', as well as twenty-five women returned as 'retired' (see Table 7.2).

Table 7.2 Occupational descriptors represented as 'nurse, not domestic servant', Edinburgh, 1861

Lady's nurse, monthly nurse	72
Sick nurse, professed nurse	97
Retired	25
RIE	61
Total	255
[Census Report: 265]	

Source: Enumerators' books, Census of Edinburgh 1861; Census Report, Scotland 1862

It seems very probable that the difference in the total between the census report and the entries in the enumerators' books represents the efforts of the census clerks to interpret some ambiguous entries. Of those women described by the single word 'nurse' in the enumerators' books, a number closely resembled those classified as 'nurse, not domestic servant' by the census

clerks. Most of the women described as 'nurse' in the enumerators' books were clearly involved principally in child care, and
of these, thirty-five closely resembled those classifed by the census
clerks as 'nurse, not domestic servant'. For the purposes of this
present study, thirty-five of the women described by the enumerators as 'nurse' have been included. In addition, three nurses who
advertised in the directory but who were assigned no occupation
by the enumerator and eleven midwives not associated with any
institution have also been included. The hospital nurses and the
retired nurses have been excluded for the purposes of this present
study, making a total study sample of 218. This sample included
seventy-four, or 51 per cent, of the nurses entered in the directory
in 1861.

A striking feature which emerged from the directories and
which was confirmed by the census was the location of the nurses'
home addresses within the city. There were distinct concentrations
in the side streets of the New Town and in the former village of
Broughton to the East. Lesser groupings existed along the routes
radiating out from the city towards the southern suburbs. All
these locations made the nurses accessible to their client groups
and to the doctors who might act as intermediaries for them. The
concentration of addresses was very specific. Some New Town side
streets only attracted one or two nurses while Jamaica Street and
India Place included eighteen and fourteen respectively in 1861
(that is, 22 per cent of all those who advertised in the directory).
The attractiveness of these streets was sustained over time.

Such a marked preference seems to demand more explanation
than simply convenient access. The social standing of India Place
and Jamaica Street was not high; the streets housed forty paupers
in receipt of relief in 1852 (all but three of the paupers were
women). By the middle of the twentieth century both were labelled as slums and demolished. It is perhaps significant that most
of the nurses resident in 1861 were either widowed or unmarried.[19] They included some older women described as retired and
some with young children. This observation could indicate that
these women had been driven to this location under the stress of
their poverty. However, the stability of this North Edinburgh
group is certainly remarkable. In no way does this group reflect
the published accounts of some observers of the urban scene in
Edinburgh who commented on the rootless and feckless habits
of the poor.[20,21,22]

On the night of the census, thirty-seven (26 per cent) of all nurses from the directory were recorded to be at work. However, of the thirty-two nurses normally resident in India Place and Jamaica Street, sixteen (50 per cent) were traced at work within the city, and a number of others were absent from home and may have been working further afield.[23] This represents an impressive employment rate and suggests that there were appreciable advantages to be gained from residence here. It may be that the patronage network involving the doctors was particularly accessible to this group of women.

The work histories of two of the women who lived here illustrate the approach which enabled some of them to pursue a successful career. Mrs Elizabeth Balmer and Mrs Mary Dearness both had rather unusual names. No one else using either name appeared in the directories at the time they were active. John Balmer, a gardener, lived in Leith between 1841 and 1851, he then disappeared and in 1853 Mrs Balmer, now living at 13 Hill Place on the South side of town appeared in all three sections of the directory listed as a 'sick nurse' in the professional directory and as a 'lady's nurse' in the street and general directories. In 1857 she moved to 10 Jamaica Street where she was still living in 1871. Her directory entries remained unchanged from 1853 to 1871. In April 1861 Mrs Balmer, a widow aged 42 was caring for the newly delivered wife of an Edinburgh lawyer in their seventeen-room home in Claremont Crescent. Such a client would have used one of the well-known doctors and would certainly have sought a competent nurse for his wife for the lying-in period. Mrs Balmer had prepared herself for this work by enrolling at the Royal Maternity Hospital in early 1851. She was there for around three months and conducted at least seven deliveries. However, she was clear about the shape she expected her career to take and only ever advertised as a 'sick nurse' or 'lady's nurse', never as a midwife. The casebook of the Maternity Hospital was not kept up continuously and the quality of recording varies; however, it is possible to trace the arrival of small groups of women described sometimes as 'midwives' and sometimes as 'pupils', at intervals of approximately three months. Mrs Dearness arrived in December 1854 at a time when the records were kept more carefully. She witnessed ten deliveries before conducting one of her own in February 1855.[24] She was rather older than Mrs Balmer and, unlike her, she appears to have begun her career while her husband Donald, an 'agent', was still alive. They both advertised their occupations from 2 Kerr Street in 1855. Following her husband's death, Mrs Dearness moved to India Place and remained there until her own death around 1870. In April 1861 Mrs Dearness, then aged 56, was also at work. She had crossed the town to the southern suburbs and was resident in the fifteen-room home of a senior Civil Service accountant. It is not clear who in the household she was caring for, but significantly, she was described simply as a 'nurse'. When at home Mrs Dearness lived with her 26-year-old daughter, a mantle maker, in a two-roomed apartment.

Both these careers demonstrate features which seem to be common to the nurses who used the directories as part of their work strategy. They were all mature women ranging in age from 30 to 74 years, the oldest nurse at work in April 1861 being Isabella Jamieson aged 68, who worked in Morningside with the 40-year-old wife of an actuary following the birth of their ninth child. Most clients appear to have conformed with the advice offered in housewives' manuals that 'a monthly nurse should be between 30 and 50 years of age'.[25] The only nurses under 30 identified in the census were working either as children's nurses in private homes or in the Royal Infirmary. Women preparing for a career as domiciliary nurses who followed the pattern demonstrated by Mrs Balmer and Mrs Dearness could only expect to find sufficient employment as mature women. The age distribution of the total sample suggests that this was indeed an important aspect of their strategy. They also needed a knowledge of the medical facilities in the city, the ability to plan and manage their time and sufficient means to support themselves and pay fees to the Maternity Hospital.[26] A reasonable standard of education would also be required.[27] Once they had gained access to the hospital, pupils had the opportunity to receive instruction from competent practitioners who also worked in private practice in the city. It was an opportunity to learn, to demonstrate personal competence and to begin building professional contacts.

Using established institutions to gain expertise and to further a career was a familiar strategy used by many individuals and all the groups seeking reform of nursing.[28] It was a strategy which acknowledged the significant skills and power perceived to be concentrated in the institutions. In the case of domiciliary nurses working with medical men who practised in both locations, it was a strategy which was calculated to optimize their opportunities for success. In order to make a reasonable living, women such as Mrs Balmer and Mrs Dearness had to strike up a satisfactory relationship not only with the patients for whom they would be caring and who paid their fees but also with those who had the medical management of the cases. Since care of post-natal women was evaluated as a particularly lucrative nursing arena, attending the Maternity Hospital, even if you only conducted one delivery, as did Mrs Dearness, gave you the opportunity to access important networks.

The social and economic success of the group can be explored when the size of the dwellings of the nurses is considered. The report of the census of Scotland for 1861 commented at length on the number of families living in single rooms. Of the entire population 34 per cent lived in one room and 37 per cent in two rooms. The figures for Edinburgh were slightly better (34 per cent in one room and 29 per cent in two rooms). Of the nurses returned as heads of households in Edinburgh in 1861, 55 per cent resided in single-room apartments, 30 per cent in two rooms, and the remainder in larger homes (see Table 7.3).[29]

Table 7.3 Size of apartments occupied by nurses identified as 'head of household'

| | Number of rooms | | | | |
	1	2	3	4	5+
Percentage of households (N = 99)	55	30	6	4	4

Source: Enumerators' books, Census of Edinburgh 1861

The significance of living in one room is possibly different for this group compared with the rest of the population. When at work a nurse was resident in someone else's home. The successful nurse was away much of the time. She might have considered it to be in her best interests to invest any excess earnings in savings rather than in a larger home.

The living arrangements of nineteen of the nurses from Jamaica Street and India Place can be discerned. This includes information relating to some of the women who were at work as their children remained at home. The number of rooms occupied by Mrs Anderson was not recorded. Of the remaining eighteen, seven lived in one room, ten in two rooms and one in three rooms, a different pattern from the total sample. Two rooms hardly represents luxury but it does indicate some degree of competence in managing resources. Several lived with their grown-up children who would also have contributed to the family income.

Of the sixteen nurses from this North Edinburgh group who were at work, three were located with their patients in lodgings in the city, and the remainder were in private houses ranging in size from seven to twenty rooms. These were primarily located in the New Town but some were also working in the suburbs to the south and north of the city. This seems to have been an elite group of patients. Mrs Junor of 16 Jamaica Street, for example, was nursing the dying Major William Blackwood in his twenty-room home in Ainslie Place. Mrs Balmer and Mrs Dearness have already been mentioned. The humblest work location of any of this group was the seven-room home of a wine merchant in Cambridge Street where Mrs Janet Spalding of 9 Jamaica Street was caring for the wife and new-born son of John Bryce.

Socially these women belonged to the respectable working class. Their children's occupations included milliner, dressmaker, 'keeps a furniture shop', pupil teacher and mariner, and several children were described as 'apprentice'. To successfully follow the working pattern they had chosen they required sufficiently polished social skills to enable them to move easily between these different worlds.

It is difficult to be confident of the extent to which the nurses were involved with each other as neighbours or fellow business-women. The apartments they occupied were within solidly built tenements and several might live on one stair. At 47 India Place, for example, lived three retired nurses aged 62, 64 and 79 years. Each returned a schedule for their own one-room apartment. Other nurses lived in similar groups in other areas of the city. Three nurses lived at 23 Howe Street, each returning their own schedule. Such arrangements, not quite living together but sufficiently closely to offer either moral or practical support may demonstrate ways in which unsupported women who wished to retain their independence and their respectability could live outside of someone else's home or an institution.

In contrast to the elite client group detailed above, some nurses were caring for patients in much humbler surroundings. Mrs Smeaton for example, who lived in Richmond Place on the south

side of town was living-in while acting as lady's nurse for the
wife of a Post Office clerk a few streets away from her home.
This family lived in three rooms with their 1-year-old daughter,
the new baby and a maid. These domestic arrangements
resembled those of some of the nurses and suggest something of
the range of social classes with whom a successful nurse would
need to interact.

So far the groups who have emerged from the data appear to
have been working as nurses. They were probably well respected
and were probably in some form of network which included the
medical establishment. They used a tool of the business world,
the Post Office directory, as part of their strategy to seek work
within that world. One group who do not emerge clearly from
the data are the midwives. Only eleven midwives were included
in the total sample, and of these, five were entered in the directory. The fate of professional midwives in Edinburgh is ambiguous. As the role of lady's nurse became more significant, that of
midwife diminished (see Tables 7.1 and 7.4).

Table 7.4 Changes in the nurse population of Edinburgh: uniquely
described as midwife

	1834	1841	1851	1861	1871
All 'nurses'	82	103	140	145	167
Midwife	46	35	28	13	5
Percentage	56	34	20	9	3

Source: Post Office directories of Edinburgh and Leith, 1834–71

On the night of the census only one midwife was recorded as
away from her own home and she was described as 'Nurse
(Midwife)' in the home of Thomas Watson, 'brass founder', whose
youngest child was already ten days old. This is not surprising if
the professional midwives served a more modest clientele who
were unlikely to be able to afford resident help for any length of
time. Their potential client group was likely to be small. Edinburgh was very well served by both doctors, attending those
with aspirations to gentility and by dispensaries. The dispensaries
served a dual purpose, offering free domiciliary care to poor
women and clinical obstetric experience to medical students and
pupil midwives.

The midwives who were recorded in the directory appear to

have constructed a lifestyle which differed from that favoured by the domiciliary nurses. Mrs Mary Anne Boyle was head in a five-roomed house in Broughton. She appeared in the directory for several years, always described as 'midwife and medical botanist'. Mrs MacKenzie at 150 High Street and Mrs Sutherland at 20 Bank Street each shared a four-roomed home with family members, some of whom were also earning. They were located in widely separate areas of the town, the latter two in the Old Town where the crowded tenements of the poor might be expected to supply a patient population for a female practitioner. Their preferred lifestyle enabled them to occupy their own larger group of rooms but at the cost of sharing a busy environment with a number of other adults. The network of supporters for this group lay within their family rather than amongst their peers.

One striking feature of both the major data sources relates to language. There is a good Scots word 'howdie' used to describe a midwife. Howdie probably equates to the English 'handywoman' but it is suggested that in the early nineteenth century howdies were trained and supported by the church.[30] Midwives working in the 1930s in Scotland spoke of them as still extant. If howdies played a role within Edinburgh they do not appear in any readily recognizable form in these records. The language used is unfalteringly English. The householders' schedules have been destroyed, and the enumerators were all educated men. As the compilation of the records moved further away from the householders they conformed increasingly to the shapes prescribed by the Registrar General.

Anne Summers considered that possibly a substantial number of the women returned as 'nurse, not domestic servant' in London in 1861 may have been independent practitioners in direct competition with the doctors.[31] This may indeed have been so in London and may hold good for some Edinburgh nurses. However, for the group examined in detail in this present study, a different work pattern seems to have been favoured. These nurses could not be described as independent practitioners who were in direct competition with doctors. Rather, they were involved in a working relationship with the doctors and an elite client group which they appear to have been able to use to their advantage. They may resemble more closely the group of private nurses welcomed by Lady Canning and described by Summers as 'lower class women who knew their place'.[32] No clear model existed which permitted women of modest means to create an independent life and at the same time to retain a respected place in the world. This chapter has suggested that a substantial group of working-class women in Edinburgh succeeded in carving out an area of work for themselves and constructed a way of living which allowed them to live as independent women. To do this they had to negotiate with and gain the confidence of the doctors and their clients. In addition they had to move back and forth physically and culturally between their own territory and that of totally different groups in society, and manage their interactions acceptably. It was his observations of the social discomfort which resulted when such skills were inadequate which inspired Dickens' portrayal of Sarah Gamp. It could be argued that to succeed, domiciliary nurses needed to acquire acceptable clinical skills and in addition to demonstrate competence in communication and in the management of their time. An important ingredient in their success may have been the support they were able to afford each other in the harsh world of nineteenth-century trade and business.

NOTES

1 C. Brontë, *Jane Eyre*, London, Penguin, 1956, p. 194.
2 A. Summers, 'The mysterious demise of Sarah Gamp: the domiciliary nurse and her detractors c. 1830–1860', *Victorian Studies*, 1989, vol. 32, no. 3, pp. 365–386.
3 C. Maggs, *The Origins of General Nursing*, London, Croom Helm, 1983, p. 31.
4 A. Summers, 'Pride and prejudice: ladies and nurses in the Crimean War', *History Workshop Journal*, 1983, vol. 16, pp. 33–56.
5 Following considerable negotiation and several abortive attempts at legislation the Medical Registration Act of 1858 ensured that all future doctors would follow a recognized professional course of study but did not forbid existing practitioners from continuing to work.
6 N. Morgan and R.H. Trainor, 'The dominant classes', in W.H. Fraser and R.J. Morris (eds), *People and Society in Scotland Vol. II 1830–1914*, Edinburgh, John Donald Publishers Ltd, 1990, p. 106.
7 This term, 'nurse, not domestic servant', used to describe one particular group of women, was first introduced in the 1861 census; however, it was never precisely defined; see: C. Davies, 'Making sense of the census in Britain and America: the changing occupational classification and the position of nurses', *Sociological Review*, 1980, vol. 28, no. 3. pp. 581–609.
8 The 1861 census was the first census which employed documentation specifically designed for use in Scotland. The census was carried out much as it is today. Schedules were distributed to individual house-

holds by enumerators who collected the completed forms on census day. Data from the completed forms were transcribed by the enumerators into their enumeration books which, in turn, were returned to Register House in Edinburgh where census clerks used specially prepared occupational dictionaries to interpret the entries in the enumeration books and compile occupational tables for the published Census Report.

9 1834 was the first year in which a 'professional directory' was included in the Post Office directory for Edinburgh.

10 R.J. Morris, 'Occupational coding, principles and examples', *Historical Social Research*, 1990, vol. 15, no. 1. pp. 3–29.

11 See, for example, Mrs Hanbury, *The Good Nurse or hints on the management of the sick and lying-in chamber and the nursery*, London, Longman, Rees, Orme, Brown and Green, 1828.

12 I. Beeton, *Household Management* (facsimile of the first edition of 1861), London, Cape, 1968.

13 Early in the century Jessy Harden commented on people coming from as far away as Belfast to consult Edinburgh doctors (see W. Park (ed.), 'Extracts from the journal of Jessy Allan, wife of John Harden' *Book of the Old Edinburgh Club*, XXX, 1959, pp. 60–118). Dr Littlejohn, Medical Officer of Health for Edinburgh from 1862 attributed the unusually high adult death rate in the salubrious New Town to the presence in those areas of 'invalids' who had come to seek medical advice (see H.D. Littlejohn, *Sanitary Report of the City of Edinburgh*, Edinburgh, 1865). The Registrar for one New Town Registration District considered that women coming to Edinburgh to deliver raised the birth rate in his District (Registrar's Notes, Quarter ended 31 March 1856, *Registrar General For Scotland Annual Reports 1855–1858*).

14 Royal College of Surgeons of Edinburgh (RCSE): Papers of J.Y. Simpson JYS 657, JYS 658, JYS 671.

15 Royal College of Physicians of Edinburgh (RCPE) Manuscript Collection: Simpson, J.Y., 17.

16 J.B. Barclay, 'John Gulland's Diary 1846–49: A transcript and commentary', *Book of the Old Edinburgh Club New Series*, vol. 2, 1992, pp. 35–115.

17 E. Vaughan (ed.), *A Victorian Edinburgh Diary: John Inglis*, Edinburgh: Ramsay Head Press, 1984, p. 58.

18 Great Britain, 'Census of Scotland 1861, Population Tables and Report': *Plt Papers (3013), L* 945, London, HMSO 1862.

19 Mrs Anderson of 28 Jamaica Street and Mrs Wilkie of 32 India Place were both at home on census night. Both were entered as 'married' and 'head' of their household which included their children but not their husbands.

20 G. Bell, *Day and Night in the Wynds of Edinburgh: Blackfriars Wynd Analysed* (facsimile of the first editions of 1849 and 1850), Wakefield, E.P. Publishing Urban History Reprints, 1973.

21 I.L. Bird, *Notes on Old Edinburgh*, Edinburgh, Edmonston and Douglas, 1869.

22 Littlejohn, op. cit.

23 Inevitably some doubt exists when identifying those at work, i.e. not at their own address. The figures cited are the most optimistic interpretation of the evidence.

24 RCPE: Edinburgh Royal Maternity Hospital: 1 Indoor Casebook 1844–1871.

25 Beeton, op. cit.

26 Fees paid by 'midwives' are recorded in the Minute Books of the Maternity Hospital. Medical Archive Centre, University of Edinburgh LHB3/1.

27 Mrs Margaret Bethune, whose ticket for the Maternity Hospital began in December 1852, purchased and used a textbook (A. Hamilton, *Concise rules for the conduct of midwives in the exercise of their profession to which is prefixed a syllabus for the use of the midwives educated at the University of Edinburgh*, Edinburgh, 1810) while in Edinburgh. She carried out her plan to return to her native village and practise. There she kept her own casebook throughout her career.

28 As early as 1840 the Institution of Nursing Sisters founded by Mrs Fry sought clinical experience in hospital for the Sisters (see A. Summers, 'The costs and benefits of caring: nursing charities, c.1830–c.1860', in J. Barry and C. Jones (eds), *Medicine and Charity Before the Welfare State*, London, Routledge, 1991, p. 133).

29 These figures are rather uncertain. The most successful and therefore the better housed nurses were likely to be absent at work and their home circumstances cannot be ascertained. Some remarkably old ladies were also included still using the title 'nurse'.

30 J. Galt, (c 1830) 'The Howdie', in I.A. Gordon (ed.), *John Galt: Selected Short Stories*, Edinburgh: Scottish Academic Press, 1978, p. 74.

31 Summers, 1989, op. cit.

32 Summers, 1983, op. cit.

Chapter 8

Ordered to care?: professionalization, gender and the language of training, 1915–37

Tom Olson

Contemporary nursing leaders have rallied around the idea of caring, claiming this as the historic core of nursing and thus the field's 'special knowledge'. This present chapter challenges the claim to caring by suggesting that caring may simply be one of several traditions that have been handed down to succeeding generations of nurses.

INTRODUCTION

This chapter aims to examine the assumption that nursing equals caring, at first glance a simple and straightforward aim. When initially presented to others, however, the responses indicated that this aim was far from simple. One prominent nurse historian suggested that I could not possibly be questioning the relationship between nursing and caring, adding that although 'you don't really say so ... I infer that what [actually] intrigues you ... [is] to spell out and verify the conflicts and tensions [around] ... being a "caring nurse"'.[1] Obviously, my point was missed – this work was not designed to verify tensions around caring but to look at the accuracy of the assumption of caring. Another nursing scholar acknowledged my intent, but insisted that to understand nursing and caring I would have to 'go back to the original source – Nightingale'.[2]

Such responses highlight the importance of this analysis, as well as the difficulty. Contemporary nursing leaders have rallied around the idea of caring, claiming this as the essence of nursing and thus the field's 'special knowledge'. Consistent with professionalization theory, identifying, developing, and successfully laying claim to special knowledge is viewed as crucial to establishing nursing as a fully-fledged profession. According to a frequently cited article in the nursing literature, 'a discipline is distinguished by a domain of inquiry that represents a shared belief among its members regarding its reason for being'.[3] Moreover, two nursing leaders assert, 'it is the common link to caring that brings nurses together'.[4] Leininger adds, 'caring is the central, dominant and unifying feature of nursing'.[5] The titles of current, well-known works in United States' nursing highlight the centrality of caring: for instance, *Care: The Essence of Nursing and Health* (Leininger 1984); *Nursing: the Philosophy and Science of Caring* (Watson 1985), and *The Primacy of Caring* (Benner and Wrubel 1989).[6,7,8]

The argument for caring is generally legitimized by asserting its historic basis. This argument typically proceeds as follows: 'Care forms the basic core of nursing actions. Traditionally, nurses have described the act of administering to patients as care behaviors.'[9] But the nurses upon whom this view is based are frequently omitted from such descriptions. In other words, caring as the essence of nursing is assumed. When nurses from the past are cited, they tend to be from the professional elite. For example, a recent article in the *Journal of Professional Nursing* quotes Isabel Stewart to underpin its warning that 'caring is slowly disappearing' from nursing. Stewart is quoted as insisting:

> The real essence of nursing ... lies not in the mechanical details of execution, not yet in the dexterity of the performer, but in the creative imagination, the sensitive spirit, and the intelligent understanding [that underlies] these techniques and skills. Without these, nursing may become a highly skilled trade, but it cannot be a profession[10]

But even in those accounts that draw on information from rank-and-file nurses, the assumption of caring remains. In one of the best known works on United States nursing history the conclusion that nurses were 'ordered to care' is reached without actually questioning the underlying premise that equates nursing and caring.[11]

In current discussions the claim to caring is often linked to feminist ideas. An article in the *American Journal of Nursing* declares that we need to value nursing, 'women's caring work', in order to 'move away from the masculine dream toward a new feminine future'.[12] From a similar point of view, the idea of 'a society that systematically undervalues care' is tied to nursing's difficulty in becoming 'a woman-valued work group'.[13] Glazer helps to clarify the gender divide that tends to frame discussions of caring. She observes that the 'view of the relative passivity of women finds a complement in feminist views of women as more cooperative and relational, more caring and less aggressive than men and ... less mechanistic and hierarchical'.[14] Caring is thus linked with passive, feminine traits. 'The "feminine" principles,' adds Passau-Buck, 'correspond to the historical roots of nursing – caring, nurturance, receptivity.'[15]

But, as one critic observes, 'if caring is really the "essence of nursing" then it must be demonstrated and not simply proclaimed'.[16] How solid is the historic relationship between caring and nursing? Was the work of nursing seen as caring, or at least something closely related to it? If not, how was nursing conceptualized?

THE RESEARCH

To explore these questions, I examined the terms and phrases used to describe nursing in the files of the 538 women who entered the St Luke's Hospital Training School for Nurses, St Paul, Minnesota, from 1915 to 1937. I focused on the 'practical records' of the programme, the collection's richest source of comments about the actual practice of nursing.[17] These records are concerned with on-the-job performance, including mastery of specific skills, and interactions with co-workers and patients. They include the observations of more than twenty-five nurses involved in supervising those in training. Interviews with several graduates of the programme were used to validate and add to this information.

On the surface, the choice of St Luke's may seem unusual. It was a well-regarded, though otherwise ordinary training programme, as perceived by community groups, accrediting agencies and prospective nurses.[18] But the ordinariness of St Luke's is exactly what makes it a useful choice. In contrast to exemplary and more typically studied schools, such as Johns Hopkins or New York Hospital, St Luke's presumably had much in common with the hundreds of other programmes that operated in hospitals across the country. During this era, those in training did most of the actual nursing work in hospitals, exchanging their labour for an apprenticeship type of learning.

The period, 1915 through to 1937, is also important in United States nursing history since it brackets the 1923 Goldmark Report, a much hailed study that was aimed at professionalizing nursing education.[19] The efforts leading up to the report were fuelled by increasing calls from nursing leaders for 'professional reform', much like that which had already occurred in medicine. As the earlier quote from Isabel Stewart suggests, these calls were remarkably similar to the rhetoric of today's nursing leaders. And yet, as noteworthy as the leaders' statements are, they do not answer questions about how nursing was perceived within the hospital, by rank-and-file nurses.

HANDLING, MANAGING AND CONTROLLING PATIENTS

One trainee, Evelyn Ferrell, was praised in 1923 as 'a good adaptable all around nurse' based on her 'way of handling patients'.[20] In fact, 'handling patients' was the phrase most frequently used to describe nursing at St Luke's. The description of Miss Ferrell is also typical in that she was referred to as a nurse, rather than as a student or student nurse, even though she was still in training.

Among the last group of women to train at St Luke's, one was described as 'a large girl – strong and capable in handling patients', and another as 'very capable in manual handling of patients'.[21] But the way in which a nurse handled patients could be a source of criticism as well as praise. For instance, a superintendent of nurses wrote to an older sister of a nurse, criticizing the younger woman's 'practical nursing'. The main problem, the superintendent explained, was that 'your sister ... find(s) it difficult to handle patients'. The superintendent added the following advice:

> [your sister] tells me that she is very much interested in English with library training, and to be very candid with you, I feel she would be more successful in this line than in nursing.[22]

Nurses frequently were evaluated in terms of how they 'controlled' and 'managed' patients also, though these terms were less commonly used than handling. For instance, a 'ward report' from 1929 described Alice Dahl as a nurse whose 'patients were always well under control'.[23] And a head nurse praised another woman in 1933 because she is 'interested in work (and) manages patients well'.[24] Other nurses received similar approval for having 'managed children well' and for having 'good control of babies'.[25]

The interviews which I conducted help to explain what was involved in handling, controlling and managing patients. Edythe Newman, a 1936 graduate, remarked, 'I don't think I'd like the nursing nowadays – it's the aides and the practical nurses who really deal with patients'. She continued, 'In those days a patient was a patient and they stayed in bed and you did everything *for* them. You gave them their bath and brought them the bed pan'.[26] Nursing in this description, 'deal(ing) with patients', means doing things for people, particularly carrying out procedures. Miss Newman was not alone in this idea.

Grace Bakke came to St Luke's from Granite Falls, Minnesota on 20 September 1928. She recorded her observations on nurses' training in several tersely worded diaries, emphasizing her first experiences involving procedures and patients, such as the following:

> 19th of November 1928, First snowfall. The first time I gave a bed bath. Gave one to Mr. Van Camp – a young flirt. I told him to finish the bath and he said he didn't need to. The sap. Complimented me to Miss Alson.[27]

Similar observations were made about 'the first time I gave a bed pan', the first 'evening toilet – made sure they [the patients] brushed their teeth and [I] gave back rubs'; the 'first enema [I] gave'; and on 4 May 1929, 'shot my first hypo'.[28] Another nurse kept a scrapbook that covered her training from 1929 to 1932. On one page is a poem that relates her experience with a patient while on night duty:

> The patient grows better night by night,
> Because some nurse in her evening plight
> Forces the fluids and forces them strong
> Keeps on forcing them all night long
> She makes drinks from oranges, from lemons, from grapes
> And Oh, what a lot of fruits it takes,
> She forces the fluid in a great many ways
> By temperature sponges, hot packs and on Trays.[29]

Like the previous examples, nursing in this situation meant assuming an assertive, vigorous role in carrying out a common procedure such as forcing fluids.

The routine of nursing is illustrated in the case records that were kept by the nurses. The two examples that follow concern patients on medical units, with undiagnosed illnesses. In the first, the work involved with one patient on the day shift is outlined:

7:15–7:30 a.m.	Feeding patient.
7:30–8:00 a.m.	Medications [given]; patient toileted.
8:00–8:30 a.m.	Patient bathed; alcohol rub; linen changed.
9:30–10:00 a.m.	Application of splint.
10:20–10:30 a.m.	Oral hygiene.
11:20–11:30 a.m.	Temperature taken.
12:20–12:45 p.m.	Feeding patient.
12:55–1:00 p.m.	Medications [given]; patient toileted; patient prepared for rest.[30]

The nurse who recorded this was working with two other patients on the same day. With the exception of the application of a splint, the list includes regularly performed tasks. In contrast, an example from the night shift lists procedures carried out in response to changes in the patient's condition:

8:45 p.m.	Vital signs taken. [Patient] complains of headache. Patient seems very excitable. Talks and laughs a great deal. Ice cap to head.
10:10 p.m.	Patient very noisy. Complains of hand feeling numb. Acts drowsy.
10:40 p.m.	[Patient] taken to Physiotherapy Room II. Drank 2 cups of water. Had difficulty in getting into bed. [Patient] complains of being cold. Extreme heat applied. Patient perspiring.
11:00 p.m.	Patient quiet and appears to be sleeping.[31]

As this shows, nursing was not simply a matter of carrying out fixed procedures, but varied depending on a patient's condition. In general, the examples suggest that handling patients involved highly physical and pragmatic actions that also required a nurse to be forceful. This impression is consistent with an era that preceded many of today's commonly used medical treatments, an era in which the main offering of hospitals was, unquestionably, nursing skill.

But nursing meant more than handling patients alone. For instance, Gertrude Rothschild was described in 1920 as 'a very capable charge nurse' for being able to 'manage both patients and doctors'.[32] This comment is noteworthy for two reasons. First, it does not seem to fit the usual view that apprenticeship stressed passivity and subservience. One of the most outspoken proponents of this view emphasizes that it was through the apprenticeship system that 'the rank and file in nursing were persuaded to believe in their inferiority'.[33] Second, the praise of Miss Rothschild stands out because it is one of the few references to physicians in the records of the St Luke's nurses. This is surprising because it has been widely assumed that 'loyalty and deference to the physician ... were stressed in hospital programs'.[34] Thus one would expect physicians to be mentioned with some regularity. In contrast, the women were more frequently evaluated on the basis of how they managed 'the helps', primarily maids and male attendants, and 'junior nurses'.[35] For instance, Florence Grant was criticized by the superintendent of nursing because 'she seemed to antagonize many of the junior nurses'. As a result, 'her associates ... did not enjoy working under her'.[36] What this information indicates is that nurses tended to function with considerable separateness from physicians. In support of this idea, Baer points out:

> Because medicine and nursing share a locus of work, a clientele group, and have certain overlapping functions, this notion of relative amounts of authority is seen as the issue when it is not the issue. ... This separateness of practice area is not, and has never been, substantially recognized.[37]

The work of the nurse was not complete with managing associates and handling patients. She was also expected to oversee the physical setting in which she worked. Thus a nurse was praised if she 'manage[d] the sick room well', 'left the ward in good condition', or 'handled [the] floor nicely'.[38] Conversely, she was criticized, as one nurse was in 1928, for leaving the 'floor in a mess'.[39] If a nurse excelled in handling patients, workers and ward, she was likely to be praised, like Elmyra Nelson, as 'an all around good nurse'.[40] Before arriving at this opinion, though, her ability to handle these areas would have been judged against the overall goal of nursing.

FINISHED WORK

At St Luke's the goal of nursing consistently focused on a tangible outcome. Handling and managing were intended to produce, in the words of the head nurses and superintendents, 'work that has a finished appearance'.[41] This phrase, more than any other, was used to gauge the women's overall success in nursing. In 1925, Alice Thompson was judged to be 'a conscientious nurse ... [because] her work presented a finished appearance and her patients were fond of her'.[42] Four years later, a Wisconsin nurse was described as 'a splendid worker ... [whose] work always looks finished ... her ward is in good condition at all times'.[43] And in 1932, Ernestine Schutt was praised for her 'neat, finished bedside nursing'.[44] On the other hand, another nurse was criticized because 'she is a slow worker and her work does not present a finished appearance'.[45]

The goal of finished work meant more than simply completing or finishing a task. Instead, it referred to the more general and observable end result of nursing work. In the diet kitchen, finished work was equated with 'serv[ing] lovely trays' and 'taking an interest in having the trays look nice'.[46] In the operating room, it meant 'keeping equipment in order and ... good condition'.[47] Overall, finished work was demonstrated by maintaining 'tidy rooms' and a 'neat ward [or floor]'.[48]

The women were evaluated in regard to their work with patients in similarly concrete terms. In the nursery, for example, 'neat, finished-appearing work' included 'keeping babies clean and dry'.[49] A nurse's work with other patients was also evaluated in regard to whether patients were clean, properly positioned, in orderly surroundings, and finally, if they 'speak well of the nurse'.[50] In general, finished work with patients meant that 'routine work ... was thoroughly completed', such as feeding, bathing and 'toileting' patients and that additional 'procedures were properly done'.[51]

To be sure, training included the practice of numerous, technical procedures that often went beyond routine tasks. Some were relatively uncomplicated, such as the preparation and collection of specimens, washing infected hair, and the administration of 'cleansing enemata'. Others required considerable skill, such as dressing burns, the use of gastrogavage, hypodermoclysis (injection of fluids into subcutaneous tissue), or bladder irrigation. These procedures epitomized the physical emphasis in nursing. To properly perform the procedures required physical strength, physical closeness and physical skill. With this emphasis it is not surprising that the aim of nursing focused on a tangible outcome: 'neat, finished appearing work.'

DISCUSSION

What is missing from the definition of nursing at St Luke's is the use of terms associated with caring, or even the term caring itself. There is no mention of words often linked to caring that were in common use during the period of study, such as nurturing, soothing and comforting. Ironically, when care was mentioned it was in reference to inanimate things, such as 'care of room or ward' or 'care of bed and bedding'. It is even more difficult to place St Luke's definition of nursing within the current rhetoric of caring. The article by Mangold, cited earlier in describing the typical argument for caring, uses the following definition of this concept and, by implication, nursing: 'assisting another to grow in a cognitive and emotional sense so that the receiver of the care may become self-actualized'[52]. In another recent example, Watson describes the aims of nursing, the philosophy and science of caring, as 'mental-spiritual growth for self and others; finding meaning in one's own existence and experiences; discovering inner power and control, and potentiating instances of transcendence and self-healing'.[53] Noddings adds that receptivity is the key to accomplishing these aims, explaining that caring occurs when the nurse 'receives the other' completely.[54]

In contrast, the women of St Luke's defined nursing as handling, managing and controlling individuals, as well as situations, with the aim of producing neat, finished-appearing work. This suggests an approach to nursing that was based in action, force and pragmatism, not receptivity. To maintain that this can be subsumed within the idea of caring threatens to enlarge this concept beyond usefulness. Consider, for instance, Reverby's description of caring: 'an unbounded act, difficult to define, even harder to control.'[55] One could argue, of course, that any comparisons between past and present descriptions of caring are invalid, as language changes over time. Clearly, the terms used to describe nursing in the past and present are unlikely to be exactly the same. Yet, if there is no resemblance in meaning then current claims to a tradition of caring are left empty. In this regard, Fischer observes that all historical questions are 'attempts to establish intelligible relationships between the signs and symbols of our language on the one hand and the evidence of our past on the other'.[56] Moreover, the work of various researchers underscores the particular importance of attention to language, past and present, in analyses involving gender and work.[57,58,59]

What then explains the marked difference between the St Luke's definition of nursing and the definitions provided in the contemporary literature? Two conclusions stand out. To begin with, the claim to caring seems to make intuitive sense, as it builds on traditional ideas of femininity. The receptive and nurturing qualities associated with caring are considered the natural domain of women generally, and nurses in particular. As a result, information to the contrary may be rejected, or at least reframed, because it does not fit with preconceived notions. As Steinberg points out, 'the central defining characteristics of jobs are often perceived in terms that are consistent with sex-role stereotypes'.[60] Steinberg takes particular note of authority, an aspect of work that seems implicit in terms such as controlling, handling and managing. She states, 'authority is part of the male sex role, and everyone sees the authority associated with male work, while the authority associated with female work is invisible'.[61] For nurses, most of whom are women, work such as handling, controlling and managing thus remains hidden, obscured by explanations that seem to have a better fit with accepted understandings of work and gender.

The belief that caring is the historic essence of nursing can also be linked to the fact that caring is identified by nursing leaders as the field's special knowledge. Porter emphasizes that 'one of the most consistent strategies to achieve professionalization for nursing has been the attempt to acquire a unique knowledge base, the possession of such knowledge being seen as one of the essential traits of a "true" profession'.[62] Caring may actually prove to be an effective rallying point for professionalization. But the findings here cast doubt on arguments that are automatically predicated upon a caring tradition. Rather than exemplifying the eternal core of nursing, caring may simply be one of several traditions that have been handed down to succeeding generations of nurses. The unquestioned reliance on caring as a distinctive point from which to analyse nursing history may cloud other meanings of nursing, particularly those in evidence among the rank and file. Indeed, the persistence of conflicting meanings or traditions may help to explain the deep divisions that continue to characterize this field in the United States, divisions that preclude agreement on even the basic issue of what preparation one must have to be a nurse.

This neither discredits the idea of caring as the goal of modern nursing nor denies that aspects of caring may be implicitly involved in nursing. Further, there is no intent to present a final answer here. Rather than frustrating the results of this particular case, however, the limitations point to additional, important questions. What might the analysis of other types of records show? What differences are suggested by focusing on caring as an ethic or attitude versus my focus, caring as nursing action? More immediately, would the St Luke's findings hold up in similar studies of other training programmes? Is it possible that caring might typify certain regions or even countries, certain periods, particular health care settings, but not others?

These questions implicitly challenge traditional ways of viewing women, as well as nursing's past. Further, as the claims to caring suggest, conceptualizations of nursing's past are at the heart of today's struggle to define the nature of nursing. The reality of this struggle is often brought to awareness in small, easily overlooked ways. For me, one reminder came during a recent visit to a prestigious university school of nursing in the eastern United States. On my way from the airport, I shared a taxi with an energetic factory nurse who lives in the same area as the university. The nurse was more than willing to share her impression of the school of nursing, though she added that she was not a baccalaureate nurse. She explained that, although the university nursing students took an impressive list of courses, the problem is that even after graduation 'they can't *control* the [hospital] unit'.

ACKNOWLEDGEMENT

The research for this chapter was supported by grants from Sigma Theta Tau International, the University of Minnesota, the

American Nurses Foundation, and the University of Hawaii at Manoa.

NOTES

1 J. Lynaugh, letter to author, 7 August 1992.
2 D. Diers, letter to author, 5 March 1992.
3 M. Newman, 'The focus of the discipline of nursing', *Advances in Nursing Science*, 1991, vol. 14, no. 1, pp. 1–6.
4 J. Lynaugh and C. Fagin, 'Nursing comes of age', *Image*, 1988, vol. 20, no. 4, pp. 184–190.
5 M. Leininger, 'Leininger's theory of nursing: cultural care diversity and universality', *Nursing Science Quarterly*, 1988, vol. 1, no. 4, pp. 152–160.
6 M. Leininger, *Care: The Essence of Nursing and Health*, Thorofare, NJ: Slack, 1984.
7 J. Watson, *Nursing: The Philosophy and Science of Caring*, Boulder, CO, Colorado Associated University Press, 1985.
8 P. Benner and J. Wrubel, *The Primacy of Caring*, Minlo Park, CA, Addison-Wesley, 1989.
9 A. Mangold, 'Senior nursing students' and professional nurses' perceptions of effective caring behaviors: a comparative study', *Journal of Nursing Education*, 1991, vol. 30, no. 3, pp. 134–139.
10 Isabel Stewart, quoted by M. Donahue, 'Inquiry, insights, and history: the spirit of nursing', *Journal of Professional Nursing*, 1991, vol. 7, no. 3, p. 149.
11 S. Reverby, *Ordered to Care: The Dilemma of American Nursing, 1850–1945*, Cambridge, Cambridge University Press, 1987.
12 S. Gordon, 'Fear of caring: the feminist paradox', *American Journal of Nursing*, 1991, vol. 91, no. 2, pp. 44–48.
13 C. Woods, 'From individual dedication to social activism: historical development of nursing professionalism', in C. Maggs (ed.), *Nursing History: The State of the Art*, Wofeboro, NH, Croom Helm, 1987, p. 158.
14 N. Glazer, ' "Between a rock and a hard place": women's professional organizations in nursing and class, racial, and ethnic inequalities', *Gender and Society*, 1991, vol. 5, no. 3, pp. 351–372.
15 S. Passau-Buck, 'Caring vs. curing: the politics of health care', in J. Muff (ed.), *Socialization, Sexism, and Stereotyping*, Prospect Heights, IL, Waveland Press, 1982, p. 203.
16 J. Morse, J. Bottorff, W. Neander and S. Solberg, 'Comparative analysis of conceptualizations and theories of caring', *Image*, 1991, vol. 23, no. 2, pp. 119–126.
17 St Luke's Hospital Training School for Nurses Collection, Boxes 1–5, Minnesota Historical Society, St Paul, MN.
18 T. Olson, 'The women of St Luke's and the evolution of nursing, 1892–1937', PhD dissertation, University of Minnesota, 1991.
19 Committee for the Study of Nursing Education, J. Goldmark,

secretary, *Nursing and Nursing Education in the United States*, New York, Macmillan, 1923.

20 St Luke's Hospital Training School for Nurses Collection, op. cit., Box 2.
21 Ibid., Box 4.
22 Ibid., Box 5.
23 Ibid., Box 3.
24 Ibid., Box 4.
25 Ibid., Boxes 4 and 3.
26 E. Newman, interview by author, tape recording, 30 December 1989.
27 G. Bakke, interview by author, tape recording, 1 April 1990.
28 Ibid.
29 H. Bertsche, interview by author, transcript and personal papers, 15 May 1990.
30 St Luke's Hospital Training School for Nurses Collection, op. cit., Box 4.
31 Ibid., Box 4.
32 St Luke's Hospital Training School for Nurses Collection, op. cit., Box 2.
33 J. Ashley, *Hospitals, Paternalism, and the Role of the Nurse*, New York: Teachers College Press, 1976, p. 84.
34 Reverby, op. cit., p. 51.
35 St Luke's Hospital Training School for Nurses Collection, op. cit., Box 5.
36 Ibid., Box 2.
37 E. Baer, 'The conflictive social ideology of American nursing: 1893, a microcosm', PhD dissertation, New York University, 1982, pp. 11–12.
38 St Luke's Hospital Training School for Nurses Collection, op. cit., Boxes 2–3.
39 Ibid., Box 3.
40 Ibid., Box 2.
41 Ibid., Box 3.
42 Ibid., Box 3.
43 Ibid., Box 3.
44 Ibid., Box 4.
45 Ibid., Box 3.
46 Ibid., Boxes 4 and 2.
47 Ibid., Box 3.
48 Ibid., Boxes 3 and 2.
49 Ibid., Box 3.
50 Ibid., Box 5.
51 Ibid., Box 4.
52 Mangold, op. cit., p. 134.
53 Watson, op. cit., p. 74.
54 N. Noddings, *Caring: A Feminine Approach to Ethics and Moral Education*, Berkeley, University of California Press, 1984, p. 30.
55 Reverby, op. cit., p. 1.
56 D. Fischer, *Historian's Fallacies: Toward a Logic of Historical Thought*, New York, Harper Colophon, 1970, p. 21.

57 A. Baron, 'Gender and history: learning from the past, looking to the future', in A. Baron (ed.), *Work Engendered: Toward a New History of American Labor*, Ithaca, NY, Cornell University Press, 1991.

58 J. Hall, 'Disorderly women: gender and labor militancy in the Appalachian south', *Journal of American History*, 1986, vol. 73, no. 2, pp. 354–382.

59 E. Faue, 'The dynamo of change: gender and solidarity in the American Labour movement of the 1930s', *Gender and History*, 1989, vol. 1, no. 2, pp. 138–158.

60 R. Steinberg, 'Social construction of skill: gender, power, and comparable worth', *Work and Occupations*, 1990, vol. 17, no. 4, pp. 449–460.

61 Ibid.

62 S. Porter, 'The poverty of professionalization: a critical analysis of strategies for the occupational advancement of nursing', *Journal of Advanced Nursing*, 1992, vol. 17, no. 6, pp. 720–726.

Chapter 9

Ambivalence about nursing's expertise: the role of a gendered holistic ideology in nursing, 1890–1990

Geertje Boschma

INTRODUCTION

A historical analysis of primary and secondary nursing literature on holism in American nursing since the late nineteenth century revealed that holistic notions which addressed the integrity and wholeness of human beings were attractive to nurses as a means of articulating their role and expertise. However, these notions also reflected nurses' ambivalence about their expertise. As a predominantly female profession, nurses struggled to define and control their specific contribution to patient care. Holistic notions of care, such as comprehensive care, patient-centred care or even total care were not merely constructs to define the professional status of nursing, but also representations of the complex and often complicated position that nursing assumed in the health care system.[1]

Major social and medical changes in the second half of the nineteenth century facilitated the development of nursing as a respected paid occupation particularly for women. Professional nursing came to be defined as a role for which a high moral standard and specific training were required. Changes in medical practice helped to make the hospital the dominant structure for health care provision. But American nursing leaders in the late nineteenth century were not concerned with hospital nursing alone. They saw nurse training in the hospital predominantly as a preparation for a more independent expert role for women in public health. From this perspective, they perceived hospital training as an inadequate preparation for the 'right breed of women' to work in public health nursing. To that end, they undertook efforts to change the educational system in such a way that it would prepare nurses for care-taking in the community. Their vision of nursing expertise was based on holistic notions of care.

However, the expanding role of nursing in public health during the early twentieth century was eclipsed by the success of hospital medicine during the 1930s. Hospital nursing became the dominant focus for the study and thought of nursing theory and practice, particularly from World War II. This shift had important consequences for nursing's perspective on holistic care. The meaning of holism changed as did its ideological function. Three shifts in the meaning of holism could be observed: holistic public health at the turn of the century, patient-centred hospital nursing in the middle of the century and the contemporary development of holistic health nursing.

The first part of the chapter examines the changes in medical thought and practice beginning in the late nineteenth century and nursing's initial focus on public health. Then the chapter addresses the shift towards hospital nursing and the explicit incorporation of holistic notions into new definitions of nursing's expertise. Within the context of hospital nursing, leaders began to define the method of nursing as a patient-centred process. Its goal was conceptualized in terms of the integrity of the individual patient. Nurses attempted to address the needs of the patient in a reciprocal interpersonal relationship promoting the patient's wholeness as a physical, psychological and spiritual being. The last section of the chapter concludes that the adoption of holistic models of care puts nursing in an ambivalent position, both from the perspective of gender and that of professionalism. Paradoxically, the patient-centred holistic approach contained a dilemma for nursing: on the one hand, nurses wanted to make the hospital a home and understand the patient in the context of his or her own life; on the other, nursing participated in a highly technocratic system that was oriented towards efficiency, organized in terms of stringent routines and always based on disembodied, specialized knowledge.

CHANGES IN MEDICAL THOUGHT AND PRACTICE

Up until the last century, medical care had been based on competing explanations of sickness. Disease was seen both as an affliction by supernatural powers and as a disturbance in the balance of natural forces that affected the equilibrium of the body or the harmony between the individual and the environment. These views changed, especially with the development of anatomy in the eighteenth and nineteenth centuries. The idea that disease could be located in specific organs and attributed to a specific cause gained momentum. With the gradual acceptance of the germ theory, the view of disease as an entity requiring a specific treatment became even more powerful. At the beginning of the twentieth century this gradually became the most widespread and accepted view of illness in the West.[2]

Nursing was one of the new professions that facilitated the acceptance of the new viewpoint at the end of the nineteenth century. Nurses brought discipline, order and efficiency into the hospitals, which were important conditions for the emerging 'discipline' of medicine to make their new antiseptic and aseptic techniques work.[3] Nurses' response to the increasing authority of medicine and the new hospital practice was ambivalent. It is the uncertainty about this change and its far-reaching implications, even today, that shaped nursing and the activities of American nursing leaders. Although the older framework of a balanced relationship between individual and environment became increasingly marginal, it seemed to provide nurses with an avenue towards adopting a more independent role. The ideals of late nineteenth-century American nursing leaders illustrated this tension. While most nurse leaders were superintendents of nurse training schools they were ambivalent about nursing's role in the hospital. Their vision of professionalism was located in the public health sphere.

AMERICAN NURSING LEADERS' FOCUS ON PUBLIC HEALTH

Dissatisfied with the fact that training appeared to mean little more than nurses being put to work as cheap labour, without any proper education for professional independence, influential nursing leaders, such as Isabel Hampton, Adelaide Nutting, as well as Annie W. Goodrich, Lillian Wald and Lavinia Dock, had other ideals in mind. Their professional aspirations were guided by a desire for self-direction and self-regulation, rather than by unquestioning obedience to authority.[4] Fascinated by the opportunities of the new public health movement and preventive medicine, their ambitions were strongly rooted in the politics of the progressive era: the feminist movement, the improvement of educational opportunities for women and social reform.[5]

The nursing leaders foresaw a new social role for nurses as health educators in the community. Although the term 'holism' was not yet used, holistic notions were applied to conceptualize the role of the public health nurse. When Lillian Wald, the famous leader in public health nursing, created visiting nursing at the Henry Street Settlement in New York, in 1893, she envisioned nursing as an all-inclusive service to patients in their homes, addressing their family situation as well as their hygienic housing and living conditions through direct care and health teaching.[6] Wald's holistic view reflects contemporary sanitarian ideas whereby improvement of living conditions and hygienic habits would bring the person into a better physical and moral state. Moreover, according to nineteenth-century morality, the nursing pioneers believed that it was their gender in particular that made women well fitted for the job. A woman had the appropriate moral influence, patience and tact to bring about changes in the lives of the citizens. Just as a mother would raise her children according to the principles of scientific hygiene, so would the nurse apply her female characteristics as a mother to the community.[7]

In order to educate nurses properly for this independent role in the community, nursing leaders sought to improve the traditional hospital training system. They perceived the apprenticeship system as insufficient preparation for providing independent social service. American leaders pleaded for improvement of education, based on their holistic perspective on the role of the nurse. By 1910 the original nursing course in hospital economics established at Teacher's College, Columbia University in New York, had evolved into a nursing department with a strong division of public service education, and was set up according to progressive ideas.[8] Nursing was conceptualized as holistic comprehensive care including physical, social and mental health aspects as well as teaching healthy living by going into the neighbourhoods, homes and schools. The education of the students was based on these notions of comprehensive care.[9]

Nevertheless, the ideal of comprehensive care was more easily incorporated in education than in practice. Initially, during the 1900s and 1910s, preventive programmes for school children, for mothers and infants, and for patients with infectious diseases, were rapidly established by voluntary agencies as well as by public health officials.[10] Soon, however, controversy arose over the various and often overlapping responsibilities of such agencies, and, more importantly, over the role of the visiting nurse. In the agencies that provided home care it was hotly debated whether sick nursing and health teaching should be performed in combination with each other or as different activities. These discussions show that already during the 1920s, ideas concerning holistic care were constrained by issues of status and specialization. Some nurses, attracted to the increased independence and status of the public health role, argued that health teaching should become a separate profession from sick nursing. In the cities voluntary and official health agencies struggled to define public health nursing. Governmental health agencies soon focused exclusively on preventive work, expecting their nurses to provide health teaching only. They did not consider bedside care, public health work. Superintendents of voluntary visiting nurse associations on the other hand argued that the combination of care and teaching was the foundation of proper public health nursing.[11] The often competing views of the public health nurses' role eventually impeded the development of a unified infrastructure for public health.[12]

While the hospital attained a central place in the health care system, the public health movement was in decline during the 1920s and 1930s. The economic depression depleted resources. Social and medical circumstances changed. The threat of infectious diseases decreased, the urban death rates dropped as did the number of immigrants, due to more restrictive immigration policies.[13] The idea of professional independence based on holistic, comprehensive care lost its community base.

'HOLISM' IN HOSPITAL NURSING

Although public health nursing declined, comprehensive notions of care did not disappear entirely. They retained an ideological function as nursing began to define its 'unique and independent expertise' in hospital nursing. As discussed above, new medical practices changed the hospital organization during the first half of the twentieth century. Gradual acceptance of the germ theory led to the introduction of aseptic and antiseptic techniques. Surgery became more successful, and the laboratory, medical science and technology grew in importance. With the growth of clinical research and with more paying patients coming into the hospital, hospital medicine was the dominant medical practice by the end of the 1930s.[14]

The growing importance of the hospital increased the need for hospital nurses. Eventually more graduate nurses became employed. Care for hospital patients became an increasingly complex and technical affair. As more surgery was undertaken, the number of acutely ill patients grew. More complicated treatment routines, observations and measurements increased demand on nurses' time and organizational skills.[15] Also, the hospital organization itself grew into a complex and bureaucratic structure. Industrial models of organization were applied in the hospital to increase its efficiency and to rationalize its organization. Consequently, nursing became more task and routine oriented.[16]

The increased significance of hospital nursing changed the focus of the nursing leadership, and reoriented their legitimation of nursing as a professional and academic discipline. The community perspective disappeared, and hospital practice became the primary focus of nursing study and thought. During the 1920s and 1930s, nursing hospital research began with time and efficiency studies applied to nursing procedures.[17] Initial enthusiasm for this type of study soon dwindled because it was too closely linked with industrial models of efficient organization, and with medical science. Such an approach, nursing leaders feared, was inconsistent with nursing's spirit and ideals.[18] Rather than focusing on techniques and the efficient performance of separate tasks, leaders began to argue that nursing needed to attend to the patient's clinical needs. Virginia Henderson, student and later faculty member at Teacher's College, Columbia University from 1931 to 1948, was probably one of the most prominent leaders to formulate this viewpoint. She introduced innovative approaches to nursing education and research and reoriented its focus towards the understanding of clinical nursing problems.[19]

Reacting against the increased rationalization of nursing practice, nursing leaders attempted to formulate nursing's *raison d'être* once again in holistic terms, but now oriented their attention towards the individual patient rather than community care, as at the beginning of the century. Hospital nursing care was redefined as a method, emphasizing the integrity or totality of the individual patient. Professional nursing methods of care delivery needed to be developed according to patient needs.[20] In order to formulate these patient-centred methods and to improve hospital care, leaders adapted previous notions of the case-study method, initially developed as a teaching tool before World War II, in the 1950s and 1960s. It was in this way that the individualized nursing care plan was developed as a model which defined nursing as a professional process or a method which was total, comprehensive and patient-centred.[21]

A pragmatic method of problem-solving was incorporated into this new definition of nursing as a process, in which the needs of the patients were identified and the nurse invited to assist the patient resolve them. Simultaneously, nursing leaders perceived this problem-solving nursing process as a psychodynamic interpersonal relationship.[22] The nurse–patient relationship was considered instrumental in resolving the patient's problems, particularly the patient's psycho-social problems, and it became incorporated within the professional definition of nursing.

Describing the task of nursing in these holistic, psychological terms represented the nurse as one who had an independent professional responsibility. Personal interaction between the nurse and the patient could contribute to the recovery of the patient. It is significant that nurses began to emphasize psycho-social needs of patients at a time when nursing was increasingly being drawn into the performance of medical techniques and assistance in medical procedures. In conceptualizing the psycho-social needs of the patient, nursing leaders attempted to identify a unique theoretical perspective on nursing study and practice; whereas medicine supposedly focused only on patients' biological needs, nursing would include patients' psycho-social needs in their care. Leaders defined the professional role of the nurse in terms of the integrity of the patient's life.

It is important to notice that these holistic notions, although they were now formulated in terms of behavioural science, were used once again to legitimize an independent expert role for nurses. The development of the holistic patient-centred approach can be seen as a professionalizing strategy with which to distinguish nursing from medicine. This distinction was a major issue for leaders of the nursing profession who sought to formulate unique theoretical frameworks for nursing during the 1960s and 1970s.

An example of one of these frameworks was the behavioural

system model of nursing, developed by Dorothy E. Johnson. Using behavioural notions such as equilibrium, stress, adaptation and system, she focused on the behaviour of the individual as a system, and considered it important that nurses perceived the person as a total organism and their behaviour as a total response. Like medicine, which focused on biological system disorders, she argued that nurses should identify behavioural system disorders, which were deviations of normal behavioural patterns. She used holistic behavioural notions as an instrument to construct a 'unique' domain of nursing knowledge and practice that was distinct from medicine.[23]

From a somewhat different perspective, but with similar holistic notions, Myra E. Levine presented a conservation model of nursing as a conceptual framework to scientifically underpin nursing practice. Whereas the goal of nursing was to promote wholeness, she argued that nursing interventions were based on the conservation of the individual patient's energy, structural, personal and social integrity.[24] Within these conceptual frameworks and within a variety of similar nursing models constructed during the 1970s, holistic care came to mean total patient care and could be used to identify the unique role of the nurse in contrast to medicine which was often represented as reductionistic.[25] Medicine, for its part, supposedly focused on disease within a biological model, whereas nursing focused on the patient's needs and his or her responses to illness. Both medical reductionism and an increasing hospital bureaucracy were criticized as objectifying patients. It was within this context that nursing saw itself as the patient's advocate and the holistic caretaker of patients.

THE AMBIVALENT NATURE OF HOLISTIC CARE MODELS

The notion of holistic care turned out to be more complicated than the nursing leaders assumed at the time. They thought that they had given a firm basis to the professional identity of the nurse. For them it was a major achievement for nursing to now be defined in relational psycho-social terms which attempted to preserve the integrity of the patient. Leaders had even designed a professional ideology to demonstrate their unique perspective in the hospital organization. And more important, they had developed a language to show that their perspective was broader than that of medicine, which was characterized in reductionistic terms valuing a 'limited' view of disease. However, this language also had a paradoxical twist. The paradoxical nature of holistic patient-centred care concepts was that their description still resonated with the older idea of nursing as a higher female calling, an idea familiar from the public health era when it was the nurse's female characteristics in particular that made her fitted for the job.[26] In emphasizing the psycho-social side of patient care, it seemed that nursing could bring into the hospital a female sphere of understanding, a particular type of emotional care that seemed to be missing in a medical, male-dominated, bureaucratic hospital system. In embracing this holistic ideology, nursing placed itself in an ambivalent position once again. On the one hand, nursing leaders had formulated a professional ideology; on the other, this new identity seemed to be repeating a pattern of making nurses, as women, responsible for bringing warmth and understanding into an allegedly dehumanized hospital. The ambiguity became even clearer as notions from the holistic health movement spilled over into holistic patient-centred models by the late 1970s.

In the 1950s and 1960s Nursing leaders had conceptualized nursing as the profession that needed to add something to the biomedical model, namely the psycho-social aspects of the care of the sick. This perspective seemed only to be strengthened, when, during the 1970s and 1980s, many notions out of the holistic health movement were incorporated into nursing.[27] The holistic health movement in the United States was a product of the counterculture of the 1960s. It proved particularly attractive to nurses.[28]

Texts such as *Holistic Nursing* by Blattner and *Holistic Health. The Art and Science of Care* by Flynn began to incorporate notions out of eastern philosophy and New Age concepts.[29] The perception of the person as a whole being, growing towards higher levels of consciousness and spirituality, in a process of self-healing and increasing self-awareness, seemed to underscore nursing's pre-existing sympathy with the integrity of the patient. A professional journal for holistic nursing and professional organizations, in particular, the American Holistic Nursing Association, were established during the 1980s to spread this new approach to nursing.[30] However, new formulations of a patient-centred perspective such as these did little to change the basic ideology. Authors who argued that holistic nursing reflected particular 'feminine ways of knowing', linked with a reflective and relational worldview underscored the dilemma, rather than providing a solution to it.[31] Those who associated nursing with supposedly feminine characteristics seemed to do little but repeat a new variation on a very old theme.

LIMITATIONS OF GENDERED, HOLISTIC NOTIONS IN NURSING

The gendered nature of holistic patient-centred approaches was exemplified by the fact that it appealed to activities such as providing empathy, warmth, love, interaction, personal care and compassion; skills that traditionally were assigned to women. This image of nursing reproduced many traditional values about womanhood: nursing as an interactive relationship, encompassing all areas of human life and intimacy. The claim that nurses' expertise was based on holistic care, therefore put nursing in an ambivalent position. On the one hand, the rhetoric would suggest that holistic nursing seemed to represent an all-embracing expertise in dealing with a person's needs and feelings. On the other hand, such an ideology was unable to address the institutional constraints and routines, the regimens of behaviour that shape the conduct of nurses and patients in the hospital. Critics such as James and Bischoff have argued that the individualized focus on the patient as a whole did not address the social context nor the organizational demands which determined the relationships between patients and nurses.[32]

In many ways the hospital structure constrained psycho-social care as much as it constrained physical care. Even in psycho-social care, nursing developed into specialized roles: on the one hand, clinical specialists were trained to deal with emotional problems in the hospital; on the other, psycho-social care persisted as an integrated part of day-to-day care and comforting activities at the bedside, which usually remained the task of less-qualified nurses or assistants. Psycho-social care was structured by a bureaucratic hospital organization. As a result, this care grew in a more complex manner than the somewhat naive holistic notions would seem to suggest. The analysis presented here reveals that nursing shifted from community-based work into an institutional structure of care provision. The institutional structure of the hospital did not diminish, but merely reproduced the existing gendered division of labour and created a hierarchical and specialized partitioning of roles and careers. The provision of emotional support or psycho-social care, quite rightly seen by nursing leaders in the 1950s and 1960s to be an important need in a growing bureaucratic hospital structure, appeared a much more complex matter than holistic nursing models were able to reveal. To simply adhere to a hollow language that resonated in only too-familiar ways with feminine identity once again put nurses in an ambivalent position and did little to promote understanding of the reality of a partial, fragmented, health care system.

CONCLUSION

Holistic notions have had an important influence upon nursing's history and ideology. However, the present analysis has argued that 'holism' as a concept was imbued with multiple meanings. It served a variety of political and ideological purposes and even had contradictory aspects. The assumption that just because women traditionally performed much of the psycho-social care, they should identify with that care and continue to do so, arguably limits our understanding of the complexity surrounding nursing's position in the health care system. Emphasizing nursing's expertise based on holistic notions provided a professional strategy with which to demand improvement of nursing education, and in the hospital context it helped nurses to establish some professional authority and independent identity. However, the strategy had its limitations. It could not be assumed that institutional hospital care, constrained by organizational routines and specialized roles, would necessarily allow nurses to perform the tasks of comforting and caring according to their personal beliefs and intentions. In the present-day context, nurses should reconsider what they mean by holistic care, what purpose it serves and how realistic it is to subscribe to it, considering the complex, fragmented institutional systems of health care within which nursing care subsists.

NOTES

1 For an overview of holistic notions of care, see C.E. Allen, 'An Analysis of the Pragmatic Consequences of Holism for Nursing', *Western Journal of Nursing Research*, 1991, vol. 13, pp. 256–72; C.E. Allen, 'Holistic Concepts and the Professionalization of Public Health

Nursing', *Public Health Nursing*, 1991, vol. 8, pp. 74–80. For a description of the diffusion of holistic ideas into nursing practice during the last two decades see M.B. Johnson, 'The Holistic Paradigm in Nursing: The Diffusion of an Innovation', *Research in Nursing & Health*, 1990, vol. 13, pp. 129–39.

2 C.E. Rosenberg, 'Florence Nightingale on Contagion: The Hospital as a Moral Universe', in C. Rosenberg (ed.), *Healing and History*, New York, Science History Publications, 1979, pp. 116–36; C.E. Rosenberg, 'Inward Vision and Outward Glance: The Shaping of the American Hospital', *Bulletin of the History of Medicine*, 1979, vol. 53, pp. 346–91; O. Temkin, *The Double Face of Janus and Other Essays in the History of Medicine*, Baltimore, Johns Hopkins University Press, 1977.

3 S.M. Reverby, *Ordered to Care. The Dilemma of American Nursing 1850–1945*, Cambridge, Cambridge University Press, 1987; C.E. Rosenberg, 'Community and Communities: The Evolution of the American Hospital', in D.E. Long and J. Golden (eds), *The American General Hospital*, Ithaca, Cornell University Press, 1989, pp. 3–17.

4 E.D. Baer, 'Nursing's Divided House – A Historical View', *Nursing Research*, 1985, vol. 34, pp. 32–8.

5 A.W. Goodrich, *The Social and Ethical Significance of Nursing*, New York, Macmillan, 1932; I.M. Stewart, *The Education of Nurses*, New York, Garland Publishing, 1950/1984.

6 L.D. Wald, *The House on Henry Street*, New York, Henry Holt, 1915.

7 K. Buhler-Wilkerson, 'Public Health Nursing: In Sickness or in Health?', *American Journal of Public Health*, 1985, vol. 75, pp. 1155–61, particularly 1157; K. Buhler-Wilkerson and S. Reverby, 'Can a Time-honored Model Solve the Dilemma of Public Health Nursing?', *American Journal of Public Health*, 1984, vol. 74, pp. 1081–2.

8 T.E. Christy, *Cornerstone for Nursing Education. A History of the Division of Nursing Education of Teachers College, Columbia University, 1899–1947*, New York, Teachers College Press, Columbia University, 1969.

9 Stewart, op. cit., p. 223.

10 Buhler-Wilkerson, op. cit., pp. 1157–58.

11 Ibid., pp. 1157–59.

12 Buhler-Wilkerson, op. cit.; Buhler-Wilkerson and Reverby, op. cit.

13 K. Buhler-Wilkerson, *False Dawn, The Rise and Decline of Public Health Nursing 1900–1930*, New York, Garland Publishing, 1989; see also Buhler-Wilkerson, 1985, op. cit., p. 1160.

14 C.E. Rosenberg, *The Care of Strangers, The Rise of America's Hospital System*, New York, Basic Books; see also Rosenberg 1987, op. cit.

15 S. Reverby, 'A Legitimate Relationship: Nursing, Hospitals and Science in the Twentieth Century', in D.E. Long and J. Golden (eds), *The American General Hospital*, Ithaca, Cornell University Press, 1989, pp. 135–56; see also Reverby 1987, p. 181.

16 See Reverby 1989, op. cit., p. 148.

17 See Reverby 1987, op. cit., pp. 144–57; Reverby 1989, op. cit., p. 142.

18 See Reverby 1987, op. cit., p. 155–6.

19 See Reverby 1989, op. cit., pp. 143–50.
20 S.R. Gortner and H. Nahm, 'An Overview of Nursing Research in the United States', *Nursing Research*, 1977, vol. 26, pp. 10–33.
21 F.G. Abdellah, I.L. Beland, A. Martin and R.V. Matheney, *Patient-Centered Approaches to Nursing*, New York, Macmillan, 1960; N. Kelly, 'Nursing Care Plans', *Nursing Outlook*, 1966, vol. 14, pp. 1–64.
22 I.J. Orlando, *The Dynamic Nurse–Patient Relationship*, New York, Putnam, 1961; H.E. Peplau *Interpersonal Relations in Nursing*, New York: Putnam, 1952; H.E. Peplau, 'What is Experiential Teaching?', *American Journal of Nursing*, 1957, 57, 7, pp. 884–6; H.E. Peplau, 'Nurse–Doctor Relationships', *Nursing Forum*, 1966, 5, 1, pp. 61–75.
23 D.E. Johnson, 'Is There an Identifiable Body of Knowledge Essential to the Development of a Generic Professional Nursing Program?, in M. Maher (ed.), *Proceedings of The First Interuniversity Faculty Work Conference*, Stowe, Vermont, New England Board of Higher Education, 19–26 June 1964; 'Theory in Nursing: Borrowed and Unique', *Nursing Research*, 1968, vol. 17, pp. 206–9; 'State of the Art of Theory Development in Nursing', in: *Theory Development: What, Why, How?* Publication No.15-1708, New York, National League for Nursing, 1978.
24 M.E. Levine, 'Holistic Nursing', *Nursing Clinics of North America*, 1971, vol. 6, pp. 253–64, particularly 258; see also 'The Pursuit of Wholeness', *The American Journal of Nursing*, 1969, vol. 69, pp. 93–8.
25 M.E. Rogers, *An Introduction to the Theoretical Basis of Nursing*, Philadelphia, F.A. Davis, 1970. For a review of holistic nursing models see J.J. Fitzpatrick and A.L. Whall, *Conceptual Models of Nursing. Analysis and Application*, 2nd edn, Norwalk, CT, Appleton & Lange, 1989.
26 C.E. Rosenberg, 'Recent Developments in the History of Nursing. A Review Article', *Sociology of Health and Illness*, 1982, vol. 4, no. 1, pp. 86–94, particularly 88.
27 R. Crawford, 'You Are Dangerous to Your Health: The Ideology and Politics of Victim Blaming', *International Journal of Health Services*, 1977, vol. 7, pp. 663–80; J.S. Lowenberg, *Caring and Responsibility: The Crossroads Between Holistic Practice and Traditional Medicine*, Philadelphia, University of Pennsylvania Press, 1989.
28 Lowenberg, op. cit.
29 B. Blattner, *Holistic Nursing*, Englewood Cliffs, N.J, Prentice-Hall, 1981; P.A. Flynn, *Holistic Health. The Art and Science of Care*, Bowie, MD, Robert J. Brady Co, 1980.
30 Johnson, op. cit., p. 136.
31 L. Kobert, and M. Folan, 'Coming of Age in Nursing. Rethinking the Philosophies Behind Holism and Nursing Process', *Nursing and Health Care*, 1990, vol. 11, pp. 308–12.
32 C. Bischoff, *Frauen in der Krankenpflege. Zur Entwicklung von Frauenrolle und Frauenberufstatigkeit in 19. Und 20. Jahrhundert*, Frankfurt am Main, Campus Verlag, 1984; N. James, 'Care = Organisation + Physical Labour + Emotional Labour', *Sociology of Health and Illness*, 1992, vol. 14, pp. 488–509.

Chapter 10

'For the benefit of mankind': Nightingale's legacy and hours of work in Australian nursing, 1868–1939

Judith Godden

INTRODUCTION

'For the benefit of mankind' is a phrase used by Elizabeth Glover, a founder of the Royal Victorian Trained Nurses' Association, in 1903. Glover responded to concern that nurses' hours of work were too long with the rebuke, 'We are professional women and work for the benefit of mankind not for twelve hours but twenty-four hours if the necessity arises'.[1]

The tone of the rebuke was not submissive but rather assertive and indignant. In this, Elizabeth Glover was not a lone or unusual voice: other senior nurses during this period similarly insisted that long hours were intrinsic to nursing. These nursing leaders actively, indignantly and consistently opposed attempts to reduce the hours of work for nurses. Why?

A starting point in understanding such opposition is to grasp the significance of the timing of the introduction of the Nightingale system of nursing. Nightingale nursing developed at a time when paid work in the public sphere was increasingly a necessary, but still highly problematic and restricted, option for middle-class women. The initial problem for Nightingale was how to legitimize nursing as a paid occupation for middle-class, lay women. Nightingale solved this initial problem by utilizing images of the nurse, not as a paid worker, but as a quasi-religious, ladylike phil-anthropist. As Baly argued, Nightingale's public relations success allowed nurses to glory in a system that resulted in high public esteem. However, initial solutions to problems became permanent as the Nightingale experiment became the Nightingale system and ossified in an atmosphere of 'obedience and conformity'.[2] This ossification occurred as a worldwide trend. Later generations of Nightingale nurses, and particularly nursing students, paid the price for retaining nineteenth-century solutions well into the twentieth century. An indication of some of the cost of such Nightingale ideals is illustrated, in the Australian context, by examining conflict over nurses' hours of work.

HOURS OF WORK

It has become axiomatic that Australian nurses have generally suffered from poor working conditions. This assumption has not always been accurate and, for example, nurses' pay has at times been relatively high for women workers.[3] However, during the century after the first generation of Nightingale nurses, there was a general recognition that nurses' living and working conditions were frequently unacceptable compared with other workers. For many nurses, working conditions declined with the severe depression of the 1890s and had not recovered by the time of the second great depression of the 1930s.

The working hours of nurses was an issue which attracted particular concern as it undermined the national image. From the 1850s, Australian workers had defended vigorously, and with some success, their right to work a maximum of eight hours a day, or forty-eight hours a week. The Eight Hour Day procession and sports day was an annual celebration, reinforcing the image of Australia as the 'working man's paradise'. Nurses who worked seventy-two hours a week undermined Australian pride in having achieved an eight-hour day for, mostly male, workers. From the 1890s, various government inquiries investigated complaints about conditions of work for nurses. Two of the more vocal were the Victorian Royal Commission into Charitable Institutions 1892–93 and the New South Wales Royal Commission into Public Charities in 1899. In addition, in 1897, the New South Wales parliament debated a motion that, 'where possible', government-employed nurses be granted a forty-eight hour working week. As one politician pointed out, women in New South Wales factories were prohibited from working longer than forty-eight hours a week. He believed that 'women [nurses] ought not to be made to work harder and longer than are men' covered by the eight-hour clauses. Another described nurses' lives as 'simply a form of white slavery'.[4] Politicians periodically voiced similar concern, such as in 1920, when Sir Joseph Carruthers in the New South Wales

Legislative Council attributed the shortage of nurses to poor pay and conditions.[5]

Feminists were also appalled at the working hours of nurses. The quotation by Glover at the beginning of this chapter was in response to the concern expressed by prominent feminist Vida Goldstein that nurses commonly worked seventy-two hours a week. In the 1930s and 1940s in New South Wales, leading feminist Jessie Street and her feminist organization, the United Associations, frequently championed the nurses' cause. In 1931, Street helped found the nurses' union in New South Wales, yet by 1944 she was complaining that nurses still frequently worked fifty-two hours a week.[6]

Newspapers and magazines provided a regular forum for complaints about nurses' working conditions.[7] One popular magazine published a particularly scathing denunciation of conditions by a reporter who temporarily became a nurse in order to write her report. The reporter contended that nursing was probably the most 'strenuous and exacting' of all women's occupations and that nurses were examples of 'sweated' labour. She called, vainly, for nurses to work only eight hours a day.[8] Women's pages of other magazines also periodically championed nurses and demanded better conditions.[9] Nursing journals, while not supporting the call for shorter hours, did allow some space for correspondents concerned about the working conditions of nurses. One such correspondent complained in 1918 that 'It is a recognised fact that the average nurse is completely run down, and sometimes quite broken in health at the end of the training'.[10]

And so the chorus of complaints about nurses' working conditions continued throughout this period.

DEFENDING WORKING HOURS

Accompanying these complaints, however, was silence. There was silence from nurses and nursing organizations in response to complaints about nurses' working conditions. In the 1897 debate in the New South Wales parliament, for example, numerous politicians opposed reducing the working hours of nurses. Some justified their opposition by insisting that nurses themselves did not want shorter hours and had never complained despite opportunities to do so. Some, including a future prime minister of Australia, William Morris Hughes, were perplexed by this lack of complaint.

Others contended that 'strong complaints ... of the long, weary hours they have to work' had been made but that nurses were not prepared to protest publicly.[11]

Some, mostly senior, nurses broke the silence but only to oppose efforts to shorten nurses' working hours. These nurses reiterated that complaints about nurses' working conditions were not legitimate. They did not stress long hours as a necessary evil, but insisted that long hours were intrinsic to good nursing. Hours that were one third longer than the community ideal were not seen as regrettable, but as desirable. Susan McGahey was Matron of (Royal) Prince Alfred Hospital, a leading Sydney hospital, and later the second president of the International Council of Nurses. She typified the uncompromising tone with her evidence in 1899 that: 'I do not consider them [nurses] to be overworked. They know when they come into the hospital what is required of them, and if they consider the work too heavy, they are at liberty to leave.'[12]

Such nursing administrators did not challenge the accuracy of the evidence cited but denied that it posed a problem. In this denial Elizabeth Glover, quoted at the beginning of this chapter, was typical. Glover was particularly indignant that would-be champions of nurses linked nurses to the campaign for an eight-hour day. Such people did 'not look upon nurses and nursing from a right standpoint. To begin with, we are not of trade, and therefore the eight hours [maximum] does not, and I hope never will, apply to nursing'.[13] It was in this context that Glover insisted that nurses were professional women who would work for the benefit of mankind all day if necessary.

Glover's objection was to nurses being associated with 'trade', and with the Australian workers' pride in the eight-hour day. The campaign to reduce nurses' working hours was dogged by this association with working-class occupations. The campaign to award government nurses a forty-eight hour week in 1897, for example, was based on the Factories Act, making nurses analogous not to high-status women but to factory workers. Glover's sentiments echoed those of the politician who, in the 1897 parliamentary debate, claimed it degraded nurses to compare them to factory hands. Similarly, a Dr Graham, in the same debate, rejected the analogy with the factory hand in favour of comparing nurses to nuns and mothers.[14]

Glover continued her rebuke by stressing that nurses were above considerations of hours of work and pay:

A nurse's life is hard, and full of self-sacrifice. . . . We must not measure our hours of labour, but rather regret that we cannot do more . . . . A good nurse can never be compensated by money. She must be paid . . . but her work must be something better, something higher, and I may add purer and holier than the ordinary commerce of today.[15]

Again, her argument was an echo of that of Dr Graham in the 1897 parliamentary debate. Whereas Reverby argued that nurses were exploited because they were primarily seen as caring in a society which devalued caring, Graham argued that nurses were more hard-headed. Nurses, in his view, accepted public esteem and an image of 'self-sacrifice and self-denial' as 'compensation' for the hardships of nursing.[16]

The issue of nursing hours again came into prominence when the labour movement revitalized the campaign for an eight-hour working day. In 1910, a number of matrons in Sydney were quoted as opposing nurses' working an eight-hour day. Not surprisingly, nurses publicly supported their leaders so that, for example, 'a chorus of nurses' on duty told a reporter that 'We don't want eight hours a day'. They claimed it was impractical and would 'upset' work.[17]

Part of the logic of the opposition to the eight-hour day was outlined by Glover in her 1903 letter. She argued that, faced with shorter hours of work by nurses, and therefore the need to employ more nurses, hospitals would not spend more on nursing salaries. Instead they would employ more nursing students who, on their graduation as nurses, would then be unemployed. This would lead to an oversupply of registered nurses which would in turn depress their salaries. Glover's attitude suggested a primary loyalty to registered nurses as opposed to student nurses, and a rigidity of thinking about hospital finances and employment opportunities for nurses.

In public, however, nurses rarely argued in terms of economic self-interest. At worst, they articulated a thin-lipped, punitive repressiveness that contemporaries labelled 'wowserism'. Such wowserism is evident in the following refusal by a nurse in 1918 to support her colleague's effort to reduce working hours:

That a nurse does not get enough sleep is most times her own
fault. You can always go to bed at 6 p.m. or 9 p.m., and once
a week you can go to bed, for instance, at 6 p.m. on Friday
and stay there till 5.30 a.m. on Sunday, if you so wish.... I
entered R.P.A. Hospital to train as a nurse, not to go to
theatres, dances and other entertainments that interfered with
my work.[18]

For such nurses, work was their prime source of fulfilment. Long
hours meant not just dedication but also busy happiness. Working
life and private life merged as all nurses under the Nightingale
system were required to be single and live in nurses' homes.
Nurses frequently developed strong emotional ties with each
other, their patients and their ward. For such nurses, nursing was
their life and they readily accepted that a 'nurse has no time for
outside interests'.[19]

During times of economic depression, the insistence on long
working hours became more exploitative as the nurses had so
little choice. Yet, it was during the 1930s depression that senior
nurses and nursing organizations stepped up their active campaign against improved working hours and conditions. At the
height of the depression in 1933, the Matron of Sydney's Royal
Prince Alfred Hospital, Miss Bossier, argued in support of an
application from Sydney Hospital that nurses should work longer
than forty-four hours a week. Bossier claimed that 'the nurse
who was interested in her work did not want too long off duty'
and that nurses had 'told her that they would rather be on
duty than have too much time off'. Working hours were not a
problem, she suggested, because nurses showed no sign of strain
and, indeed, were often 'exuberant' in the nurses' home, and
even frequently danced after duty.[20]

In the 1930s one of Australia's leading nursing organizations
was the Australasian Trained Nurses' Association (ATNA).
ATNA lobbied hard to prevent a reduction in working hours and
to prevent an increase in nurses' salaries. The executive argued,
like Glover in 1903, that shortened hours would 'inevitably' lead
to more nursing probationers and would 'overcrowd the market
with nurses': 'To shorten hours and increase salaries will naturally
add to the attractions of the profession .... One of the declared
objects of the Association has been to devise some scheme to
decrease the supply of trained nurses.'[21]

If this argument is to be taken at face value then this must be one of the few cases where a professional organization tried to improve working conditions by making the occupation so unattractive as to, even in a major depression, deter its own practitioners from working! That ATNA was controlled by doctors increases suspicion about the validity of the arguments put forward. Doctors and nurses employed by the same hospital and health care system were, after all, competing for their share of the same pool of money.

Registered nurses, however, were also competing against unregistered nurses, the nursing students. Hospitals, as is evident from the arguments of ATNA, were perceived as considering that nursing students could frequently be substituted for qualified nurses. Senior nurses in ATNA accepted this view and did not campaign to limit the nursing role of students. Instead they propagated a mystical view of all nurses having common interests and being above campaigning to improve their working conditions. Why?

Part of the answer can be found in the underlying economic arguments mentioned above. Other explanations include: the lack of alternative occupations for middle-class (and aspiring middle-class) women; the influence of military discipline and ideals; the demand by hospitals (including private hospitals owned by nurses) for cheap labour; the influences of the religious nursing orders; and the domination of nursing by the medical profession. Part of the answer can also be found in the initial compromises Nightingale made in order to achieve acceptance and status for female nurses working in the public sphere. It is this aspect which is explored in the rest of this chapter.

NIGHTINGALE'S COMPROMISES

Florence Nightingale dominated and shaped general nursing from her time in the Crimean War (1854–56) onwards. She was responsible for a radical change in the image, and to a lesser extent the reality, of nursing. This change of image was from that of a drunken, callous, old, working-class 'Sarah Gamp' to that of a young, middle-class, idealistic nurse.[22]

Australian colonists shared the determination to improve the standard of nursing and they too looked to Nightingale. The Nightingale Fund responded to an appeal from Henry Parkes, the New South Wales Premier, and sent a Lady Superintendent and five nurses to Sydney in 1868. Lucy Osburn, the Lady Superintendent, was expected to administer nursing at Sydney Infirmary and also to train nurses who would spread the Nightingale system of nursing throughout the Australian colonies.[23] The eagerness with which Australians welcomed Nightingale nurses, and with which Osburn propagated the Nightingale system until her retirement in 1884, has been outlined elsewhere.[24]

When Nightingale and Osburn were reshaping nursing, paid work in the public sphere was increasingly a necessary, but highly problematic and restricted, option for middle-class women. Both Nightingale and Osburn had only one model of high-status, lay, middle-class women working in the public sphere. This model was that of organized philanthropy by elite and middle-class women, an activity which was widespread both in England and Australia.[25] Philanthropy organized by women was publicly acknowledged as an important part of the social welfare system of the Victorian age. There was no other public work by lay women that carried as high a status but the catch was that philanthropy was unpaid, voluntary work. Nurses under the Nightingale system needed to be paid in order to attract sufficient numbers of women willing to submit to the rigours of training. In addition, it was assumed that working-class women needed to be supervised by middle-class women. Therefore, nursing needed middle-class managers, nursing 'sisters'. The problem was that such middle-class women lost status by earning a salary. When 'ladies', from need or preference, worked for a living, they were recast as 'gentlewomen', to denote their loss of status.

Nightingale paved the way for acceptance of nursing as an appropriate occupation for lay women by claiming that nursing was part of the woman's sphere and by allowing a class-based nursing hierarchy.[26] Her trump card, however, was linking nursing to altruism – to the high status of philanthropic ladies such as Nightingale herself, and to the religious vocation of the nursing nuns. While Nightingale nurses had to be trained and paid, their motivation to undertake nursing was to be similar to that of a religiously inspired vocation. Nightingale won the right for middle-class women to work in the public sphere but only by obscuring the essential nature of nursing as an occupation and a means of earning a living. Nightingale was successful precisely because her system was seen as meeting contemporary expectations regarding the need for training, for a class-based hierarchy, and women working only from a philanthropic motivation. The Nightingale system meant 'paid well-trained Nurses ... under the immediate supervision and guidance of ladies who undertake the duties of Sisters from the highest and purest motives of benevolence'.[27]

Nursing was a paid occupation for women, but was constructed as a religiously inspired philanthropic vocation. This very uneasy compromise bore with it the fundamental resistance of nurses to the notion that they shared common interests with other workers. As the Nightingale 'system' ossified, many nurses had to be content with public esteem rather than material reward. In particular, long hours of work became intrinsic to the values of Nightingale nurses and a symbol of their altruistic motivation.

NURSING MOTIVATION

Charitable motivation was at the heart of Nightingale nursing. Nurses trained at St Thomas' Hospital under the Nightingale Fund were bonded to work for four years in a charitable institution, that is, a public hospital or workhouse infirmary. Nightingale nurses were discouraged from undertaking the often more lucrative and congenial private nursing. As Nightingale wrote, '*in none of our Training Institutions*, have we anything to do with training nurses for the *rich – or sending out women to nurse at home*'.[28] Private nursing of wealthy patients could not be disguised as charity; it placed individuals outside the control of a female head; and, if the Nightingale nurses were treated like domestic servants, threatened to undermine their newly won, idealized status. Accordingly, Nightingale insisted that a gentlewoman was ennobled by nursing in a hospital ward, but degraded by nursing rich and especially male, patients: 'A young gentlewoman lowers herself by nursing young gentlemen or noblemen – not her brothers – except in War or Epidemics.'[29] Similarly in Sydney, Lucy Osburn wrote caustically about nurses who left to undertake private nursing, one of whom did so by trying to disguise her intention.[30]

Nightingale's stress on charity and religion as nursing motives increased as she realized how far the myth of the success of the Nightingale Fund fell short of its actual achievements. Nightingale received warnings about the poor state of the Nightingale School of Nursing from 1871.[31] By 1873, Nightingale advised that the Fund had to lie to the public and that Mrs Wardroper's management of the Nightingale School was disastrous. Nightingale wrote that Wardroper was 'more of a slave-driver & less of a woman every day ... not ... capable of any considered opinion or judgment ... utterly impracticable, inconsiderate, untrustworthy, forgetful', unable to tell 'a sheep's head from a carrot', accepting incompetent sisters and illiterate nurses, and maintaining her power through a 'spy system' and a 'petty, irreligious, Boarding School' spirit. Wardroper agreed with Nightingale that the School of Nursing was 'falling to pieces' and that 'gentlewomen' were refusing to stay. Nightingale was distressed that probationers in the School established in her name underwent 'no training', but did 'nothing but make beds & empty slops' and that their 'so very severe' work and inadequate diet resulted in high levels of sickness.[32]

Nightingale would not, or could not, do much to improve conditions. Instead she urged the probationers to endure their conditions and not to reveal the discrepancy with the public image. To achieve her ends, Nightingale increasingly exploited religious and philanthropic ideals. Privately, Nightingale was extremely sceptical about the authority wielded by churches.[33] Her private doubts, however, did not lessen her insistence that nursing be done through a Christian motivation. In her annual addresses to probationers, religious motivation was constantly stressed. Nurses were dichotomized into 'good' and 'bad' nurses and religious authority used to enforce high standards of nursing care and obedience. In 1872 she stated her belief that the 'first and most important question for each of us Nurses' was 'Am I a Christian?' The following year she promoted Christianity as a means of preventing nurses becoming 'hard' or 'shallow'. In 1874, nurses were urged to be 'missionaries for good', and to live 'for God'. The following year they were told that Christ was 'our example and pattern'. By 1900 Christ was the 'author of our profession' and probationers honoured or dishonoured him through their nursing.[34]

Religion was only one of the sources of pressure on nurses to conform as the problems of management within the Nightingale School intensified. Nightingale became increasingly adept at invoking all means of ensuring she commanded respect and obedience. The onus was increasingly placed on the nurses to prove that their motivation lived up to the Nightingale ideal. In 1873, women were to nurse from higher motives, not the 'mere scramble for remunerative place'. By 1883 Nightingale admonished nurses for having other than 'high' motives; nurses' 'calling' was to alleviate suffering, 'not to amuse ourselves'. Nurses were to have 'moral motives' and their ward work should be 'thorough and perfect'.[35]

The stress on self-abnegation, in response to the chaos of the Nightingale School, was strengthened with each year. The yearly addresses to the Nightingale nurses illustrate the pressure to conform. In 1874, the probationers were told that the 'highest exercise [is] self-denial ... without it [will come] the ruin of the nursing'. In 1875, Nightingale scolded the nurses, telling them that they had a 'great name' in the world but only 'for conceit'. The Nightingale Fund, she assured them, did not want any woman who questioned any aspect of the Nightingale system. Probationers were 'not to question so much'; they were taught to 'reason why' but not to reject the information. They were cared for 'as if you were our children', and 'self-esteem' was nominated, along with a 'domineering temper', as the two great temptations to avoid. By 1876 nurses who complained were 'Pharisees'. In 1878 they had no 'business' and it was 'so cowardly to complain'. The next year, Nightingale demanded four qualities from her nurses: comradeship, discipline, humility and obedience. By 1881 they were told they came to be taught, and were urged to accept their teaching with 'gentleness, patience, endurance, [and] for-bearance [sic]'.[36] There were to be limits on their learning; Nightingale urged the probationers to be good rather than clever nurses.[37]

As Nightingale attempted to conceal the disaster at St Thomas's School of Nursing, the concept of nursing as a vocation, far removed from considerations of working conditions, became irrevocably linked with the Nightingale system. This identification was confirmed by the so-called Nightingale pledge, written by an American nurse in 1893 and repeated by generations of hospital trained nursing students in Australia, England and elsewhere. With this pledge each nursing neophyte 'solemnly pledge[ed]' before God to be a good woman ('to pass my life in purity') and a good nurse ('to practise my profession faithfully'). The pledging nurse publicly identified nursing with loyally 'aid[ing] the physician in his work', with an added commitment to 'devote myself to the welfare of those committed to my care'. In Australia, politicians, hospital administrators and doctors were all too ready to stress that hospital nursing was not so much an occupation as an act of charity.[38]

The cost of that act of charity, however, fell more heavily on some nurses than others. At the beginning of the Nightingale experiment, the work and interests of the 'lady supervisors' were distinct from that of the bulk of the nursing workforce. During the twentieth century, these distinct interests were preserved between the supervising sisters and the nursing students. The division of interest within nursing was based on the great irony that most of the nursing workforce were nursing students, not qualified nurses. Nursing students were the only members of the nursing staff to be called 'nurse', but they were the only ones who were not 'nurses', at least in the legal sense of being registered nurses. In addition, during this century most nursing students were young. They were vulnerable and their relative powerlessness resulted in longer hours than those worked by their seniors. For example, in 1933 at Sydney's Royal Prince Alfred Hospital, nursing students worked an average of 52.5 hours a week, while sisters worked an average of 48 hours.[39]

CONCLUSION

This chapter took as its starting point Elizabeth Glover's opposition to shortening nurses' long working hours at the turn of the century. Senior nurses such as Glover insistently and continually denied that long hours were a problem for nurses. This chapter has explored why such an attitude to nurses' working hours prevailed, as well as the ways in which influential figures attempted to justify it. The premiss has been that this attitude was a logical extension of Nightingale's arguments when she first tried to legitimize, then salvage, the Nightingale system of nursing in the 1870s. Under the Nightingale system, long hours became a symbol of dedication over and above that of the usual worker. Long hours were seen as excluding potential nurses lacking the necessary strength, single-mindedness and/or dedication. Long hours and poor conditions made those nurses who remained 'special' and gave nursing an idealized status.

The tragedy for nursing is that the Nightingale legacy was multifaceted and had the potential to change. Nightingale became increasingly maudlin in old age but she also always advocated that nurses never cease to learn and adapt their ideas. Contrary to popular myth, for example, Nightingale did embrace the new ideas of antisepsis and asepsis.[40] Yet Nightingale's initial compromises ossified into a rigid system that was resistant to change. Her desperate attempts to paper over the cracks at St Thomas's became the Nightingale system. Nurses who accepted the idealized Nightingale image saw themselves as elevated above the mundane concerns of other workers. They had no defence against long hours and poor working conditions. Nursing students, who undertook most of the bedside nursing, were the most vulnerable and worked the longest hours. If Nightingale nursing was a quasireligious, charitable act, then the long hours worked by the nursing students simply highlighted the essence of nursing. How could hours of work be relevant when the aim was 'the benefit of mankind'?

ACKNOWLEDGEMENT

My thanks to the Wellcome Institute for the History of Medicine for a grant which enabled me to consult the Nightingale papers.

NOTES

1 E. Glover, letter to editor, *UNA, Journal of Nursing*, 1903, vol. 1, p. 11.
2 M. Baly, *Florence Nightingale and the Nursing Legacy*, London, Croom Helm, 1986, p. 222.
3 J. Castle, 'The development of professional nursing in New South Wales', in C. Maggs (ed.), *Nursing History: The State of the Art*, Beckenham, Croom Helm, 1987.
4 M. Cordia, *Nurses at Little Bay*, Prince Henry Hospital Trained Nurses' Association, Sydney, pp. 46, 25, 41.
5 *Sydney Morning Herald*, 19 November 1920, p. 9c 'Plea for Nurses'.
6 J. Godden, 'The unionisation of nurses', in H. Radi (ed.), *Jessie Street. Documents and Essays*, Sydney, Women's Redress Press, 1990.
7 For example, *Sydney Morning Herald*, 25 November 1910, p. 8, 26 January 1912, p. 3.
8 B. Tracey, 'The Ministering Angel', *The Lone Hand*, III:15, 1 July 1908, pp. 236–42.
9 For example, *Town and Country*, 10 December 1930, p. 8.
10 *The Australasian Nurses' Journal*, 15 October 1918, pp. 344–5.
11 Cordia, op. cit., pp. 31, 33, 39, 43, 45, 40–1.

12 S. McGahey, Royal Commission into Public Charities, Evidence, *NSW Legislative Assembly Votes & Proceedings*, 1899, p. 60.
13 Glover, op. cit., p. 11.
14 Cordia, op. cit., pp. 24–5, 34–5, 39.
15 Glover, op. cit., p. 11.
16 Cordia, op. cit., p. 34.
17 *Sydney Morning Herald*, 25 November 1910, p. 8.
18 *The Australasian Nurses' Journal*, 16 September 1918, p. 307.
19 Ibid., 16 December 1912, p. 416.
20 *Sydney Morning Herald*, 29 June 1933.
21 Australasian Trained Nurses' Association (ATNA) folder titled Formation of NSWNA, MLMSS 4144.
22 See especially, C. Davies (ed.) *Rewriting Nursing History*, Croom Helm, Beckenham, 1980; and R. Dingwall, A. M. Rafferty, and C. Webster, *An Introduction to the Social History of Nursing*, Routledge, London, 1988.
23 F. Nightingale to Sir H. Verney, 16 April 1867, Wellcome Institute mss folder for 1867.
24 J. Godden, 'Victorian influences on the development of a professional identity with nursing', in G. Gray and R. Pratt, *Scholarship in the Discipline of Nursing*, Melbourne, Churchill Livingstone, 1995.
25 F.K. Prochaska, *Women and Philanthropy in 19th Century England*, Oxford, Oxford University Press, 1980; J. Godden, 'Philanthropy and the woman's sphere', PhD thesis, Macquarie University (NSW, Australia), 1983.
26 Godden, 1995, op. cit.
27 Medical Committee, A Statement by the Middlesex Hospital, December 1865, BLMS 45752, f.125.
28 F. Nightingale to E. Verney, 13 July 1871, BL ADD MSS 45802, f.233. Emphasis in the original.
29 F. Nightingale to H. Bonham Carter, 23 February 1873, f.267, BL ADD MSS 47717.
30 L. Osburn, Nurse Register, Sydney Infirmary, 1868–84, pp. 34, 54.
31 F. Nightingale to H. Bonham Carter, 24 June 1871, BL ADD MSS 47716, f.202.
32 Ibid., 23 February 1873, f.268, BL MSS ADD 47717 and 8 October 1873, f.219 BL MSS ADD 47718; [17 or 18 January 1873], f.184, 188; 9 February 1873, f.238, 249–51; BL MSS 47717; 28 February 1873, f.69, 8 October 1873, f208, BL MSS ADD 47718 and 23 February 1873, f.268, BL ADD MSS 47717; 22 April 1873, f.9, BL MSS ADD 47718; [early 1872], f.195; [17 or 18 January 1873], f.196–226 BL ADD MSS 47717.
33 F. Nightingale to Sir Harry Verney, 25 December 1866, Wellcome Institute, folder for 1866.
34 F. Nightingale, Address to Probationers, August 1872, p. 8; 23 May 1873, p. 8; 1874, p. 9; 1875, p. 6 GLPRO, MSS HI/ST/NTS/CL3 and 28 May 1900, MSS 5476/119, Wellcome Institute.
35 F. Nightingale to H. Bonham Carter [1873], BL ADD MSS 47717,

f.27; F. Nightingale, Address to Probationers, 1883, p. 8 and 1886, p. 13. GLPRO, MS HI/ST/NTS/CL3.

36 Ibid., p. 2; 1879, p. 3; 1872, p. 2; 1874, p. 8; 1875, pp. 4, 5–6, 11; 1878, p. 9; 1879, pp. 1–2; 1881, p. 12.

37 Ibid., 1881, p. 12 cf. Charles Kingsley's famous line, 'Be good, sweet maid, and let who will be clever'.

38 For example, Cordia, op. cit., p. 43 and S. Forsyth, 'Professionalism and nursing', Masters thesis, University of Sydney, 1994, p. 103.

39 *Sydney Morning Herald*, 29 June 1933.

40 L. Wilson, letter, 13 May 1876, GLPRO, HI/ST/NTS/Y/17; F. Nightingale, Address to Probationers, 1897, p. 3, GLPRO, MS HI/ST/NTS/CL3.

Chapter 11

Employment conditions for nurses in Australia during World War II

Glenda Strachan

'The remuneration now paid to qualified nurses is so inadequate that to secure their future they must leave the profession.'

The 1939–45 war posed a direct threat to Australia. The war in the Pacific reached the shores of Australia with the bombing of Darwin in February 1942 and the sinking of the hospital ship *Centaur* on 14 May 1943 when it was a mere forty miles east of Brisbane with the loss of 268 lives, including eleven of the twelve nurses aboard.[1] Nursing, as a major provider of health care, held an essential place on the policy agenda during World War II. The demands of a nation at war and the needs of the civilian population, the changes in working conditions and the position of women in the workforce, had profound effects on the nursing labour force. The period was characterized by extreme shortages of nurses caused by the demand for nurses from the military services and the increased competition for employment from other occupations and industries at home. As the threat of an invasion of Australia intensified in 1942 and the requirements of the armed forces and war-supply industries increased, women's labour became indispensable for the war effort. Women entered industries in which they had not worked previously and took up jobs which had previously been unacceptable, although these were usually semi-skilled jobs. The Australian government's approach to this crisis of insufficient labour was to enter the names of women on to a register with a view to encouraging them to work in essential industries or in the female branches of the forces. When encouragement failed to provide suitable distribution of this labour, force in the form of direction orders was used. In Britain too, forms of compulsion were used to enhance the distribution of women's labour and from 1943 all nurses were obliged to obtain employment through the Ministry of Labour and National Service. Recruitment campaigns which were organized on a voluntary basis, however, were confined to Canada.[2]

The problems of the distribution of women's labour were compounded by the disparity of women's wages and working conditions. Women were attracted to better paid 'war work', new areas of employment which had emerged to meet wartime demands. Other work in which women had traditionally been employed, such as nursing and clothing manufacture, had great difficulty attracting women because they retained lower rates of pay and poor conditions. Government inquiries into nursing shortages noted that nursing suffered by comparison with other occupations open to women but no national attempts were made to readjust nurses' wages.

The government's response to the problems in the distribution of female labour during the war, including the shortage of nurses and hospital domestic staff, was one which relied on direction to move women to areas where their labour was needed. Many workplaces, including hospitals, were designated as protected undertakings and the rights of employers and employees were limited, including the right of the employee to leave the job and of the employer to dismiss a worker.[3] Direction to specified work was the final method of control, with failure to follow orders resulting in an appearance at a magistrate's court and possible fine. The engagement of labour was so severely circumscribed by the manpower regulations that Mr Wallace C. Wurth, Director-General of Manpower in the Ministry of Labour and National Service, characterized the situation as coming very close to total civilian conscription for industry of those regarded as available labour – married women with dependants, for instance, were excluded.[4]

While it was clear that encouragement in the form of better working conditions produced results, this was not employed as a strategy for remedying the problems. As shortages of workers increased and women's protests over their low pay in certain industries heightened, the government was forced to reassess women's wages and some workers received pay increases. This did not affect nurses and indeed exacerbated the problem. The health industry experienced such severe problems that the Acting Commonwealth Statistician reported that 'hospital staffs were so short as to seriously embarrass provision of hospital services'.[5] The Manpower Directorate, in charge of the movement of labour, concentrated on direction rather than encouragement through offering better wages and conditions. Government records do not leave any clue as to why this was not tried. Rather than encouraging women to enter hospital work through better pay and conditions, government regulations forced women to work in hospitals and fined those who did not comply with these orders. Why did the authorities not concentrate on improving the lot of the nurse? Was it a belief that the only true nurse was one who did not care about her own well-being or retirement income, that nursing demanded self-sacrifice in a way that other occupations did not?[6] The fact that nursing was treated differently to other occupations may suggest this, but the decision-making criteria used by government committees are not made explicit.

SHORTAGES OF NURSES

Shortages of nurses were evident by the latter half of 1940 and during the war numerous government committees investigated the situation and presented similar findings.[7] At a 1941 conference the Country Hospitals Association, representing seven hospitals, stated that they continued functioning only 'by the overworking of the Hospitals' permanent staff. In some instances, nurses, after having worked twelve hours a day have to attend urgent operations at night'. The secretary of the association feared that 'constant overwork at high tension' was 'not likely to endure, and we feel ere long, the nurses who are bearing "the heat and burden of the Day" will succumb to their labour'. The conference concluded that the immediate remedy was a revision of the rates of pay for nurses by the hospitals but the Australian government took no immediate steps.[8] In August 1942 a government committee investigating nursing concluded that:

> a major cause of the shortage of nurses for civilian requirements is the inadequate salaries paid to nurses in public hospitals and other institutions requiring the services of nurses. Civilian nurses' pay compared unfavourably with that of

nurses in the services and most unfavourably with the pay ruling for other occupations in which women were engaged.[9]

The committee believed that the government should intervene to increase nurses' salaries but these recommendations were not followed. There was, nevertheless, widespread community agreement that nurses' conditions needed improvement. The *Cairns Post*, a regional newspaper, commented that:

Nursing is an arduous profession, but it carries with it great responsibilities, irregular and long hours, and a certain amount of danger from infection. The reason why so many girls go in for it is because, generally speaking, they are idealists, who wish to serve unfortunate people who are suffering in health. Because of this idealism they are likely to be made use of, for they are loath to fight for their rights like other classes of the community.[10]

Miss C.E. Nell Grant, matron of a small county hospital, wrote in the *Australasian Nurses' Journal* that it was not surprising that young women were not taking up nursing. The situation was likely to continue for as long as 'girls can obtain employment in more lucrative professions where they are not required to do night duty nor work so strenuously, and have week-ends and public holidays off'.[11] A few lone voices suggested that the remedy lay in actually giving better conditions to nurses. In federal parliament Senator McLeay commented on the 'alarming' situation in November 1944:

Why is the shortage of nurses so acute? One reason is that whilst the Government apparently is prepared to go to any length to improve working conditions in munitions factories, it is not willing to take similar action to improve the conditions of nurses who spend many years in training and engage in laborious work for many hours each day. The Government eventually will be forced ... to ensure that the remuneration of nurses shall be more comparable with that of women working in munitions factories and in other attractive avenues of employment.[12]

Nell Grant was more specific in her proposals for change, suggesting eight-hour rosters for nurses.[13] Higher salaries and better conditions for nurses were not implemented. Compulsion was chosen instead. In January 1943 legal and administrative control of nurses passed to the Manpower Directorate which assumed full responsibility for the control of all nurses and hospital staff.[14] While voluntary transfers to hospital work were encouraged, the powers of direction were used to direct 'nursing personnel into positions where they would be best able to utilise their nursing qualifications and as the public interest demanded'. On 3 June 1943 Wurth instructed his deputies that sufficient opportunity had been given for nurses and domestics to come forward voluntarily and, 'after a well-publicised final appeal, steps should be taken to direct single women to hospital work'. Direction to employment in hospitals was included in the almost 10,000 direction orders issued between August 1943 and July 1944.[15]

At times the situation was so desperate that patients were refused admission and denied urgently needed treatment because of staff shortages. In June 1944 the shortage of nurses (including trainees) in civilian hospitals was assessed at almost 1,300 and in addition nurses were needed for work in private homes, welfare work and government departments, and the services were forced to release women for civilian hospital employment. Part of the problem was a 'marked decrease' in the number of trainee nurses who provided extensive labour in hospital wards. Securing adequate numbers of trainee nurses was a complex issue because there were so many avenues of employment open to young women. Publicity campaigns, or 'active propaganda' as Wurth described it, were mounted in the press, on radio and in films. The shortage of nurses was compounded by a shortage of domestic staff in hospitals which was itself 'largely due to problems of differential wages, and generally the more favourable opportunities in industry for women'. In order to conserve scarce resources, trained nurses were requested not to perform domestic duties, an order which was impossible to follow in most hospitals.[16]

NURSING CONDITIONS IN QUEENSLAND

The extent of nursing shortages made conditions very onerous in some hospitals, especially those in country areas. In the state of Queensland, for example, some hospitals were so short-staffed that nurses threatened to take or took strike action in an effort to exert pressure on the authorities to improve their conditions.

The picture of docile, compliant, obedient servants of the hospitals taking such drastic action was out of character with their tradition and training but conditions became so difficult that nurses decided to take this step. Industrial action was not limited to nurses. Reekie argues that in wartime conditions:

> there was ample opportunity for resistance to develop from blatant wage injustices, the widespread introduction of shiftwork, the use of new and sometimes hazardous materials, insufficient amenities for workers in industry and clear anomalies between conditions in the 'war' industries and those in traditionally female occupations.[17]

In Queensland, nurses' strikes in 1944 and 1945 resulted from problems of low staffing levels and poor working and living conditions as the nurses endeavoured to pressure the authorities into providing more staff. Women 'felt so strongly about injustices suffered in the workplace that they dared defy a community consensus that there be no strikes in wartime'. In this way 'women's militancy... challenged the image presented in the media of the contented, patriotic female war worker'.[18] Such actions were all the more extraordinary when taken by the traditional carers of the community, nurses, who had absorbed the tradition of sacrifice to a high degree.

On 2 August 1944, thirty trainee nurses at Cairns Hospital in north Queensland went on strike for the day without consulting or informing their trade union, the Australasian Trained Nurses' Association (ATNA). They complained of the 'excessive hours, overdue holidays, food conditions, lack of cutlery, ward utensils and no lounge in which to entertain friends' as well as an acute shortage of staff. The hospital needed an additional nineteen trainee nurses and six domestic staff.[19] After a lengthy conference with hospital board members and officials of the local Trades and Labour Council, they resumed work on the condition that their demands were met within a week.[20] Manpower authorities combed the local area for young women enticing them to become trainee nurses and appealing to 'parents, employees and other persons likely in any way to influence any eligible young women, to do nothing to prejudice their taking up this urgent and essential hospital work'.[21] The local president of the Country Women's Association asked her members to help in recruiting nurses:

We know that one does need to be of the necessary temperament to be a success; but there are many girls most suited for this profession, good, healthy Australians filled with the milk of human kindness. Will you try to convince your friends with growing girls that one of them at least might consider nursing as a career? The noblest of any![22]

But the acute nursing shortage that persisted meant that two hospital wards remained closed. One hundred young women were interviewed by manpower staff but only three volunteered as nursing trainees and four were appointed as domestics. Eighteen direction orders were issued by the manpower authorities, sixteen for nursing trainees and two for domestic staff. Only four women started work, but this number was offset by two nurses wanting to leave work because they were getting married. Despite all these efforts and the dire step of industrial action by the trainee nurses, there was a net gain of only eight nurses by the end of August 1944.[23]

Mental hospitals also suffered acute problems. A shortage of seventy nurses at the Goodna Mental Hospital in south-eastern Queensland led to a five-day strike by female nurses. Mr F.E. Walsh, Deputy Director-General of Manpower in Queensland, reported that 'owing to staff shortages, the nurses employed had been carrying on under great strain and now felt that they could not continue this much longer'.[24] But manpower authorities were unsuccessful in their attempts to find additional nurses and by 18 April the male nursing staff of 170 threatened to strike with the female nurses if the situation could not be alleviated. Fifty-five additional workers including twenty-five army nurses and four volunteers were obtained to begin work at the hospital and Walsh threatened to prosecute women who disobeyed direction orders without a satisfactory excuse.[25] In the same month staff at the Willowburn Mental Hospital at Toowoomba, south-eastern Queensland, threatened to strike and manpower authorities hastily directed women to this work.[26] Shortages of nurses persisted and in March 1945 sixty-one nurses at Willowburn Mental Hospital stopped work, requesting twenty-one additional nurses. Manpower authorities responded by directing young women to this work.[27]

Other hospitals and health services were affected and country towns supported nurses who were attempting to preserve health services in their communities. In April 1944, when manpower authorities suggested that the Gin Gin and Mt Perry Hospitals in central Queensland should be closed, the local shires protested vehemently.[28] When the Collinsville District Hospital in north Queensland experienced difficulties, the coal miners in this town and nearby Scottville threatened to strike in sympathy with the overworked nurses, as they were 'determined to exert pressure on the authorities to see that the hospitals are adequately manned'.[29]

Manpower authorities did not have much success in directing women to hospital work for conditions remained poor, and women were discouraged by the fact that once they accepted work in a hospital they were forced to remain there by the wartime regulations. Force was used in the form of prosecutions to draw women into hospital work. For instance, the Brisbane Summons Court fined one woman five pounds, with two pounds eight shillings costs, or in default three weeks' imprisonment, for not reporting to the Goodna Mental Hospital on 7 April 1944. Another woman, who had treated the direction order 'with some contempt', according to the magistrate, was also fined.[30]

NURSES' SALARIES

It was obvious and freely admitted that the problems of staffing hospitals related to the unattractiveness of the employment. The first meeting of the Central Nursing Sub-Committee in 1942 had identified the inadequacy of nurses' salaries as the reason for the shortage and decided that it should attempt to secure an increase in pay for nurses. But there were difficulties in adjusting the rates of pay for, while the central sub-committee could make recommendations to the Minister, the Minister could give effect to them only by regulations under the National Security Act. This would have been relatively easy if the rates of pay for nurses had varied slightly from state to state, but the difference in salaries was great, especially for trainees. The Central Nursing Sub-Committee faced a dilemma. Unification of trained and trainee nurses' salaries at the highest level would involve extra expenditure of approximately £200,000 to £250,000 annually. A further difficulty was that there was no uniform rate of pay for nurses in the states of South Australia and Tasmania.

While the federal government enacted specific legislation using its defence powers to raise other women workers' wages, this route was not followed in the case of nurses. The 1942 sub-committee suggested that the nurses' association, the ATNA (registered as a trade union in some states), should use federal industrial relations legislation to apply for increased wages through a federal award.[31] Although the federal government had established an Arbitration Court, its power to set wages was circumscribed by the Australian Constitution (in comparison, state governments faced no such limitations) and this route would have taken many years and probably been unsuccessful because of these constitutional limitations.[32] The suggestion of this form of federal regulation showed a lack of industrial knowledge on the part of the committee. Moves for a federal award did not proceed yet this goal meant that other means of securing changes were not pursued vigorously. Because of the difficulty in remedying the wide discrepancies in salaries from state to state, the problem of central regulation of salaries was set aside. The only alternative left was for salary changes to occur on a state basis. For instance, it was not until late 1943 that there was any change in the nurses' award in Queensland. The dire shortages prompted the ATNA to approach the court for an increase in wages. The association argued that over 800 trained nurses in Queensland had left the profession and sought employment in other more remunerative areas of commerce, arguments that were substantiated by most of the employers. Reasonably attractive salaries needed to be offered to retain an adequate staff of nurses and induce new trainees to enter the profession and the Brisbane and South Coast Hospitals Board, the largest in the state, even proposed a scale of increased salaries.[33] While higher rates of pay were granted they still left nurses financially behind other workers. A staff nurse earned three pounds a week (plus board and lodging) after completing a four-year apprenticeship while a female shop assistant earned three pounds, ten shillings. A female clerk earned four pounds, four shillings and six pence per week.[34] As well as the low remuneration in relation to the nurse's skill and experience, nurses' working week was four hours longer than that prescribed for most other workers. Women workers, of course, earned substantially less than men, and although there was a wide variety of wage rates for women during the war, women's wages averaged only 59.5 per cent of male wages in 1943.[35]

Wage rates clearly had an affect on the distribution of female labour. A 1941 survey of 800 women commencing work in a munitions factory revealed that some women 'wanted to do something to help the war effort: but, if questioned directly, the majority admitted that the relatively high wages had also affected their decision'. Many could earn more than twice their previous wage in the munitions factory and thirty-eight or nearly 5 per cent of this sample had been nurses.[36] This increased competition with other occupations had disastrous consequences for the staffing of hospitals. The differences in rates of pay for women, from the low pre-war rates in traditionally female jobs and industries to the equal pay awarded in a few areas, created major problems in the distribution of female labour. A specific Women's Employment Board (WEB) operated from September 1942 until October 1944 to fix the remuneration, hours and working conditions in newly created wartime jobs and work women did which released men for other military or civilian jobs.[37] Although WEB decisions affected only 9 per cent of the female workforce, it usually awarded 90 per cent of the male rate. However, the state and federal industrial tribunals continued to arbitrate on the wages and working conditions of other women workers such as nurses, using the traditional criteria which had kept women's wages at about 55 per cent of the male rate.[38] The wide disparity in women's wages, exacerbated by WEB decisions, gave rise to a great deal of discontent among women working outside war industries and those who had been employed in munitions work before the war. Low wages and the disparity of wages in traditional female industries led to strikes of women workers, particularly among textile workers.[39] Women wanted jobs at the higher WEB rate. Despite the government's direction powers, women deserted low-paid jobs when they could to take up the war work which paid 90 per cent of the male wage. Wurth himself stated:

> obviously, women have been attracted into the higher wage occupations rather than into the low ones . . . . Of course, other motives besides the opportunity for earning attractive wages have induced many women to offer themselves for employment, but the influence of higher wages was probably the most significant.[40]

By 1943 the federal Arbitration Court was forced to award 75 per cent to women in the clothing and rubber industries in an effort to keep them at work.[41] This serious problem led to a re-examination of the position of women's wages and in August 1945, as the war ended, the National Security Regulations provided that the remuneration of women in vital industries should not be less than 75 per cent of the corresponding male rate.[42] Although a severe shortage of both domestic staff and nurses in hospitals was acknowledged, these regulations applied to hospital domestic staff but not to nurses.[43] The increase in the wages of the domestic staff upset the relativities of the female staff in hospital employment and left nurses' wages further behind those of other workers. There was no satisfactory resolution of the question of the regulation of nurses' wages and no steps were taken to encourage more women to work in hospitals or train as nurses. Instead, the remedy was authoritarian.

RECOMMENDATIONS FOR SOLVING THE NURSE SHORTAGE

In January 1945 a committee was appointed by the Minister for Defence to enquire into the shortage of nurses to serve the civilian population.[44] The committee's report was submitted on 4 June 1945, a month after Germany had surrendered in Europe but two months before the war in the Pacific ended.[45] Yet again the thrust of the report was that the pay and conditions for nurses were totally inadequate. The committee emphasized that all the evidence supported the view that there would not only be no improvement in the nursing situation in Australia, but that the position would deteriorate rapidly unless all federal and state governments were prepared immediately to vastly improve the rates of pay for all classes of nursing, conditions under which nurses lived and nursing education.

The evidence that the committee took from trainees and trained nurses was that salaries were 'hopelessly inadequate'. It believed that 'the remuneration now paid to qualified nurses is so inadequate that to secure their future they must leave the profession'.[46] In fact the committee:

> came across instances where prospective trainees went out to work in other occupations in an endeavour to secure sufficient money to enable them to enter the nursing profession, and in all the lower paid States the trainees frequently said that they

could not live without parental assistance on the wages they received during their training period.[47]

Some trainees were earning as little as fourteen shillings per week, leaving eleven shillings after tax had been deducted. There were great discrepancies in the amounts deducted for living allowances and 'in view of the appalling staff accommodation seen in a number of hospitals it would appear that there is little justification for the amounts deducted'. The committee commented that 'under such circumstances, the causes of discontent are self-evident'. Because of the policy of utilizing trainees as a form of cheap labour, too much of the nurse's time was taken up in domestic work. Now that there were more avenues of work open to women at much better rates of pay, many young women chose this over a life, at least in the short term, of poverty and restriction. Once again, in the face of three years of nursing shortage, the basic problem of low pay for nurses exacerbated by the increasing competition from higher paid jobs for women, was identified as the major problem.

Looking to the future, the 1945 government committee did not feel that there would necessarily be a sufficient number of nurses when the war ended:

because during the war tens of thousands of young women have been living under better conditions .... From the Committee's investigations nothing was heard to indicate that when the war ends any of these young women are likely to enter nursing. At the present rates of pay and conditions Service personnel are receiving, they regard a nursing career as economic retrogression.[48]

The committee concluded that 'the shortage of nurses cannot be improved until the nursing profession is made worthwhile to the trainee and trained nurse, and until conditions become sufficiently attractive to hold suitable trainees, and likewise, to hold the nurse when she has qualified'. Shortly after this report the war ended and the nurse shortage question ceased to be a national issue and was left to the field of state regulation. Several committees with senior personnel had deliberated for many years over the problems of staffing hospitals during the war. The solution was seen as better pay and conditions for nurses but recommendations which actually achieved this were not forthcoming.

So what was so disconcerting about raising nurses' wages or giving them better working conditions, especially since this was acknowledged as the cause of the shortages? Increased nurses' wages would have added considerably to the cost of running hospitals and this could have been a significant disincentive. Were the authorities afraid of equal pay with its implication of giving women an equal place in society or recognition that their labour was equal in worth to that of men? The composition of the various committees, with senior medical and nursing personnel, may have led to an acceptance of the place that nurses held within the hospital hierarchy. Better pay could have disturbed this relativity. In addition, the practical problems in implementing these changes were complex. Difficulties of state and federal regulation of pay and wartime wage regulations meant that a simple solution could not be found. But in other occupations the federal government had legislated to increase the rate of pay.

In July 1944 Major-General S.R. Burston, Director-General of Medical Services, noted:

> the pay of munition workers, clerks and stenographers, in fact almost any class of work open to women, is better than nursing and when the long period of training, the poor pay, compared to the high degree of professional responsibility a nurse must accept are taken into account, it is not surprising that the supply of trainees is not equal to the demand.[49]

Thus it was acknowledged at the highest levels that nurses were among the women workers worst off in terms of their wages and conditions. Instead of enticement in the form of better conditions, force was used in an attempt to staff hospitals adequately. Powers of direction were used, often without the desired result. Never was it contemplated that the dire labour shortages could be handled by raising nurses' wages so that they no longer needed to leave the profession to secure their future or to create a career structure that would turn nursing into a credible alternative to the 'professions' that commentators continued to perceive as rivals.

NOTES

1 R. Goodman, *Queensland Nurses: Boer War to Vietnam*, Boolarong, Brisbane, 1985, p. 207.
2 P. Summerfield, *Women Workers in the Second World War*, Rout-

ledge, London, 1984, pp. 31–7; R. Pierson, *'They're Still Women After All': The Second World War and Canadian Womanhood*, McClelland & Stewart, Toronto, 1986, pp. 22–61.

3 W. Wurth, *Control of Manpower in Australia: A General Review of the Administration of the Man-Power Directorate February, 1942–September, 1944*, Government Printer, Sydney, c. 1944, pp. 71–85.

4 Ibid., pp. 107–10.

5 Ibid., p. 390.

6 See G. Strachan, 'Sacred Office, Trade or Profession? The Dilemma of Nurses' Involvement in Industrial Activities in Queensland, 1900 to 1950', *Labour History*, 1991, no. 61, pp. 147–63.

7 New South Wales MCC to CMCC, 17 Oct. 1941; Department of Health; Reports of the Central Medical Co-ordination Committee 1938–Feb 1946; 'Nurses General File' 1941–1942: CP94/1, item 0134/7/26, Australian Archives, ACT.

8 Report of proceedings of conference held for the purpose of discussing difficulties experienced in hospital management owing to the shortage of nurses, 26 Sept. 1941. Department of Defence III General Correspondence (Unclassified) Series 'O' Multiple Number System: 'Control of Nurses', 1942–1943: A663, item 0130/1/731, Australian Archives, ACT.

9 Sir Alan Newton, Deputy Chairman CMCC to all Deputy Chairmen, 5 Aug. 1942; Department of Health Central Medical Co-ordination Committee General Correspondence 1939–1945, 'Nurses Co-ordination' 1942: CP432/2, item bundle 3, Australian Archives, ACT.

10 'Melbourne Letter: Nurses' Salaries', *Cairns Post*, 7 Aug. 1944.

11 C. Grant, 'Annual Meeting, Queensland', *Australasian Nurses' Journal*, June 1945, p. 84.

12 *Commonwealth Parliamentary Debates*, vol. 180, 1944, p. 2429.

13 Grant, op. cit., p. 84.

14 W.C. Wurth, Director-General Man-Power Directorate to Deputy Directors General, 26 Jan. 1943; Department of Defence III General Correspondence (Unclassified), Series 'O' Multiple Number System 'Control of Nurses' 1942–1943: A663, item 0130/1/731, Australian Archives, ACT.

15 Wurth, op. cit., pp. 97–9, 178–80.

16 Wurth, op. cit., pp. 177, 180; S. Butlin and C. Schedvin, *War Economy 1942–1945*, Australian War Memorial, Canberra, 1977, p. 374; W.C. Wurth to Deputy Director-General, 10 Apr. and 18 Aug. 1943; W.C. Wurth to all Deputy Directors General, 21 Sep. and 6 Oct. 1943; Department of Labour and National Service Correspondence: B550, Australian Archives, Victoria; W.C. Wurth to Secretary Department of Defence, 20 June 1944; Department of Defence III General Correspondence (Unclassified) Series 'O' Multiple Number System ('Medical Manpower – Services and Civilian Requirements') 1944: A663, item 0130/1/791, Australian Archives, ACT; 'Stalwarts of Australia's Hospitals', Australian *Women's Weekly*, 8 Apr. 1944.

17 G. Reekie, 'Industrial Action by Women Workers in Western Australia during World War II', *Labour History*, 1985, no. 49, p. 82.

18 Ibid., p. 81.
19 List of Strikes in Queensland for month of August 1944; Department of Labour and National Service, Central Office; General Correspondence of the Secretariat, and Administrative and Industrial Relations Divisions, 1940–c.1950: MP574/1, item 420/1/18, Australian Archives, Victoria.
20 'Trainees Strike', *Cairns Post*, 2 Aug. 1944.
21 'Securing Hospital Staff', *Cairns Post*, 3 Aug. 1944.
22 'M. Christina Atherton to editor', *Cairns Post*, 8 Aug. 1944.
23 'Hospital Staff', *Cairns Post*, 8 Aug. and 10 Aug. 1944; 'Closing of Wards', *Cairns Post*, 29 Aug. 1944.
24 'Urgent need', *Queensland Times*, 11 Apr. 1944.
25 'Nurses Threaten Strike', *Queensland Times*, 8 Apr. 1944; 'Urgent Need', *Queensland Times*, 11 Apr. 1944; 'Goodna Strike', *Queensland Times*, 17 Apr. and 19 Apr. 1944.
26 'Strike Threatened', *Queensland Times*, 28 Apr. 1944.
27 'Nurses Stop Work To-Day', *Courier-Mail*, 21 Mar. 1945; '243 Patients Unattended', *Courier-Mail*, 22 Mar. 1945; 'Girls Ordered to Willowburn', *Courier-Mail*, 23 Mar. 1945.
28 'Closure of Hospitals', *Queensland Times*, 22 Apr. 1944.
29 'Nurses Threaten to Strike', *Queensland Times*, 27 Apr. 1944.
30 'Two Women Fined', *Queensland Times*, 29 Apr. 1944.
31 Control of the Nursing Profession Memorandum by Dr J.H.L. Cumpston, Director-General of the Emergency Medical Service, 16 Oct. 1942; Department of Health Central Medical Co-ordination Committee, General Correspondence 1939–1945 'Nurses Co-ordination' 1942: CP432/2, item bundle 3, Australian Archives, ACT.
32 Section 51 (xxxv) of the Constitution gives the federal government its major industrial relations powers and allows this government to legislate for 'the prevention and settlement of industrial disputes which extend beyond the boundaries of any one state'. Until 1983 the High Court interpreted the meaning of 'industry' in a way which limited it to production and associated areas such as banking. Teachers and firefighters, for example, were not able to gain a federal award because they did not work in an 'industry', with the result that these groups were restricted to operating under state industrial legislation. It is likely that any attempt to gain a federal award by nurses would have been challenged successfully in the High Court. (P. Punch, *Guidebook to Australian Industrial Law*, 4th edn, CCH, Sydney, 1984, pp. 19–21).
33 *Queensland Government Gazette*, 1943, vol. CLXI, no. 71, 8 Sept.
34 Ibid., no. 27, 2 Aug. 1943.
35 Calculated from weighted average nominal weekly rates. Commonwealth Bureau of Census and Statistics, *Labour Report 1947*, Commonwealth Bureau of Census and Statistics, Canberra, pp. 58, 60.
36 H. Crisp, 'Women in Munitions', *Australian Quarterly*, 1941, vol. 13, no. 3, pp. 72–3.
37 P. Hasluck, *The Government and the People 1942–1945*, Australian War Memorial, Canberra, 1970, pp. 266–7.

38 E. Ryan and A. Conlon, *Gentle Invaders: Australian Women at Work*, 2nd edn, Penguin, Melbourne, 1989, p. 136; K. Darian-Smith, *On the Home Front: Melbourne in Wartime 1939–1945*, Oxford University Press, Melbourne, 1990, p. 64; M. McMurchy, M. Oliver and J. Thornley, *For Love or Money: A Pictorial History of Women and Work in Australia*, Penguin, Melbourne, 1983, p. 111.
39 McMurphy, Oliver and Thornley, op. cit., p. 113.
40 Wurth, op. cit., p. 162.
41 McMurchy, Oliver and Thornley, op. cit., p. 112.
42 Ryan and Conlon, op. cit., pp. 133–4.
43 National Security (Female Minimum Rates) Regulations, Statutory Rule no 139, 1945 and *Commonwealth Gazette*, no. 170, 4 Sept. 1945.
44 Preliminary Report of Committee Appointed by the Minister for Defence, 5 May 1945; Department of Defence III Correspondence File Multiple Number System (Class 301) (Classified), 'Medical Manpower Position in Relation to the Services & Civilian Needs – Statement by Services Medical Directors' 1943–1946: A816, item 11/301/552, Australian Archives, ACT.
45 Report of Committee Appointed by the Minister for Defence, 4 June 1945, ibid.
46 S.R. Burston, Major-General D.G.M.S., to Director-General of Manpower, 24 July 1944; Department of Defence III Correspondence File Multiple Number System (Class 301) (Classified), 'Medical Manpower Position in Relation to the Services & Civilian Needs – Statement by Services Medical Directors' 1943–1946: A816, item 11/301/552, Australian Archives, ACT.
47 Ibid.
48 Report of committee appointed by the Minister for Defence, 4 June 1945, ibid.
49 S.R. Burston, Major-General D.G.M.S., to Director-General of Manpower, 24 July 1944, ibid.

Chapter 12

Seeking jurisdiction: a sociological perspective on Rockefeller Foundation activities in nursing in the 1920s

Sarah Elise Abrams

The literature on professions and the process of professionalization has sometimes distorted our perceptions of the power of professions and their relations to the clients they serve. Older models of professions such as the model proposed by Carr-Saunders and Wilson in the 1930s, and those proposed by Miller-son and Wilensky respectively in the 1960s, focused on such attributes as possession of an esoteric body of knowledge, extensive training, self-regulation and service commitment.[1] Friedson challenged prevailing ideas by suggesting that autonomy, rather than organization or training, distinguished a true profession in an evolving world.[2] Sociologist Andrew Abbott has, more recently, taken a systems approach to how professions are constituted and how they behave in social contexts.[3] Abbott's theory of the system of professions is helpful in explaining various forces that shape occupations in the current health care system. The extent to which Abbott's model also affords a framework against which to examine the early twentieth-century attempt of nurse reformers to professionalize the occupation is the subject of this chapter.

The process of achieving control and professional legitimacy as described by Abbott is illustrated in events related to Rockefeller Foundation (RF) support for medicine, public health, social work and nursing during the period of 1915 to 1930. Medicine and public health activities in the RF have been well documented but, until recently, Foundation contributions to nursing have received scant attention. The story of the waxing and waning of RF interest in American nursing illustrates the possibilities and constraints faced by aspiring professions during the early part of this century.

WORK, KNOWLEDGE AND LEGITIMACY

Although Abbott theorizes about the internal and external dynamics of recognized professions, only a few concepts that are particularly relevant to historical events in nursing are presented here. Abbott's concept of jurisdiction provides a basis for analysis of the meaning and authority of professions. He proposes that professions gain and retain power through a claim to *jurisdiction*, a legitimate sphere of authority in which not only the nature of work but that of expert knowledge is defined and controlled. *Legitimacy* is achieved in a dynamic process involving public perceptions and policies, legal authorities and constraints, power and competition.

Abbott addresses fundamental questions about the evolution of professions and the interrelationships among them, and he proposes some ways that occupational groups control knowledge and skill. Professions are distinguished from other occupations in Abbott's system by the control of a body of abstract knowledge out of which grows practical application. Crafts or skilled occupations, on the other hand, control primarily technique, or application. Although techniques and applications in the professions may be delegated to others, abstraction is retained by those identified as the professionals. Abbott argues:

> Only a knowledge system governed by abstractions can redefine its problems and tasks, defend them from interlopers, and seize new problems – as medicine has recently seized alcoholism, mental illness, hyperactivity in children, obesity, and numerous other things. Abstraction enables survival in the competitive system of professions.[4]

Nightingale's reform efforts provide Abbott with an example of the competitive nature of professional jurisdiction. In his view, nursing represents a 'classic case of limited settlement' within the jurisdictional area of medicine. Nursing's settlement was achieved by subordination; that is, even though Nightingale envisioned a profession that had parity with medicine, with independent authority and specialized training, her vision was unacceptable to the border sentries of medicine.[5] Medicine absorbed incursions at the borders of its territory by redefining the problems with which it was concerned and negotiating subordinate limited settlements with competitors who posed a threat to medicine's defined jurisdiction. Thus, leaders of the medical community could argue successfully, for a time, that custodial care in, and the administration of, hospitals were tasks subordinate to the medical care given in them. The issue is one of relative control. No profession ever has exclusive control over knowledge or work. The scope of medical authority, like that of other professions, is granted by public policy and legal action. These, in turn, are influenced by power, prestige and the ability of one or another profession to control access to knowledge to the extent of making it inaccessible to potential interlopers.

One historical dilemma in viewing the subordination of nursing to medicine is the issue of how nursing gained occupational status. In contrast to Abbott, Friedson had argued that nurses, in order to gain an entree to the hospital, deliberately subordinated their work to that of medicine, thus assuring a limited, 'semi-professional' status for the occupation.[6] Whether either medicine or nursing based practice on abstract knowledge or technical application was, at best, arguable during the early part of the century. The question of autonomy, too, left room for debate. Private duty nursing was perceived as either domestic in character or else subject to the dictates of physician orders. Nurses functioning outside the hospital environment were, however, probably less constrained than their hospital-based peers in setting the standards for and controlling the performance of nursing work. Conclusions about the subordination of nursing as an occupation and its possession of at least certain of the attributes of other professions during the time period are not absolute.

Abbott suggested that jurisdiction may be enclosed or seized by a group that comes into existence for a particular purpose. This occurs only rarely and only when dominant individuals or organizations direct the process.[7] Nightingale, an individual with sufficient personal charisma and power to accomplish this feat, laid the foundations for nursing's control of its own work. The impact was minimal, though, because nursing care was not a significant area of work for the dominant profession of medicine.[8] Conflict began to develop when nursing practice began to encroach on areas previously exclusively within medicine's jurisdiction. Philanthropically supported reform efforts illustrate how redefinition of nursing jurisdiction through the creation of formal educational systems and control over its work was attempted.

THE INFLUENCE OF THE ROCKEFELLER FOUNDATION

Early corporate philanthropy had a profound impact on nursing, mainly by giving nursing issues a place on their agenda – a form of legitimacy rarely granted to nursing before this time. The RF was officially chartered in 1913, and prominent nurses were beginning to discover that private charitable foundations might offer the means to achieve some of the goals towards which they had been working for the previous twenty years. The Rockefeller Foundation contributed little to nursing during the Foundation's formative period, but by the 1920s, RF interests and the agenda of selected nurse leaders converged, if only briefly. Between 1918 and 1930, the RF donated $2.3 million to a variety of nursing projects, studies and institutions in the United States. In total, between 1918 and 1954, the Foundation expended only $5.8 million on nursing education projects worldwide, and another $7 million on nursing activities not related to schools of nursing.[9] Although these contributions were nominal compared to the Rockefeller Foundation funds for medicine and public health, the monies nevertheless helped nursing through a difficult developmental period by establishing educational models, supporting public health nursing demonstrations, and perhaps most important, by fostering the growth of an international network of nurse leaders who worked to advance the interests of the profession throughout the course of the century. Whether the Foundation's choices of projects and individuals to support were essentially benign – selection of the best offered – or whether they were meant to spread an economic ideology and support a class structure through the medium of a professional class has been debated for over a decade.[10] The politics of RF action can certainly be argued, but there is no question that a broad impact was felt in nursing.

AMBIGUITY AND AMBIVALENCE

The position of the RF regarding the actual work of nursing or the attempts of its occupational leaders to gain professional recognition was, however, historically ambivalent. There were a number of reasons why this was the case. Nursing's subordinate status in the medical and public health activities of the

Foundation accounts for some inconsistencies in approach. But there were other factors unrelated to nursing which precipitated the waxing and waning of interest in nursing. Within the Foundation itself dissension about who would control which fields of activity affected nursing's location in the various units of the organization. The Rockefeller Boards were autonomous, a consequence of having been formed at different times and for distinct purposes. The historical evolution of the Boards often led to duplication, conflict and confusion, not only among Foundation staff, but also in the minds of Foundation beneficiaries and the public.[11] Individual officials of the Rockefeller Foundation also had specific interests of their own to promote – public health, education, research, and social experimentation. Proponents of each of these interests viewed nursing from a different perspective, and rarely as a separate field of Foundation interest. Recognizing this, the question is whether nursing can be regarded, as Abbott suggests, as merely a case of limited settlement within medicine's legitimate jurisdiction.

RF officers issued formal and informal statements about policies related to nursing between 1915 and 1930. Interest in nursing as a field of practical activity was first stimulated by the public health and social reform movements and the shortage of qualified nurses occasioned by World War I. By 1925, educational projects in American nursing had been subordinated to international public health interests as well as the demands of both domestic and international medical education. During a conference in October 1925, RF future intentions towards nursing were articulated.[12] The agreement between selected officers specified that emphasis would be placed on preparing leaders, not 'rank and file' nurses, through 'cooperative' efforts designed to create or strengthen institutions to serve as 'lighthouses' or models for replication.

The involvement of the RF in funding nursing proposals was at least partly due to the support of Edwin R. Embree, hired as secretary of the Rockefeller Foundation in 1917, and director of the Division of Studies, effective 1923. In both capacities, he had the primary responsibility for nursing education activities in the United States between 1918 and 1928. Annie Warburton Goodrich, Dean of the Yale School of Nursing considered him a great supporter.[13] Previously uninitiated about nursing work, his education was largely directed by Lillian Wald and Goodrich who were at the Henry Street Settlement during the early years of Embree's involvement. There were those, however, including Foundation officers and nurses, who perceived Embree as confused and promoting goals that were inconsistent with the professional agenda of recognized leaders in nursing. His own views of nursing were necessarily affected by the inconsistencies in position exhibited by nursing leaders, of course, but Embree also held opinions about the behaviour of nurse leaders with respect to other nurses. His support of F. Elisabeth Crowell, the RF director of nursing activities in the Paris Office, put him at odds with American nurse reformers who perceived Crowell negatively. Embree was also put off by the arguments among nurses about education and the control of subordinate personnel. Nurses criticized, perhaps because they did not feel that Embree was representing their case as well as he might. They may also have resented their reliance on him, knowing that they had no other voice promoting the professionalization of nursing in the Foundation. As a result, Embree was stung by the criticism from the very individuals whose causes he had helped to promote within the Foundation.[14]

The problem was, in part, that Embree showed greater concern for social reform than for professionalization and did not agree fundamentally with the choices and compromises made by American nurse reformers. He argued that nurse leaders confused what he considered the 'simple issue of education' by arguments over the duration of coursework and practical training and the status of other workers.[15] His personal records do not give any indication, though, that he opposed nursing's efforts to gain either academic status or independence from the hospital. Embree might have taken a more consistent approach in presenting programmes to the RF Board of Directors had nurse reformers defined the boundaries of professional nursing more clearly themselves. Even after a decade of immersion in nursing issues, Embree wrote about nursing as one mystified by the persistent lack of clarity about it.

Actually, Embree was not alone. Ambiguity about nursing's jurisdiction, that is, its exclusive and legitimate knowledge and work, preceded the involvement of the RF. In 1911, Adelaide Nutting, America's premier proponent of nursing education that was not dependent upon hospital support, had applied to the Carnegie Foundation on behalf of the ASSTS to fund a study of nursing education similar to Flexner's evaluation of American medical education.[16] The Flexner report, one of a series under-written by the Carnegie Foundation, was a detailed analysis of medical education that ultimately resulted in the closure of many substandard schools throughout the United States. Henry S. Pritchett, Carnegie's chairman, possibly hoping to deter Nutting, asked what the function of the nurse was. Not content to leave her choices completely open, he questioned whether nurses were fitted 'to analyze and deal with the phenomena of disease', or were simply 'trained with the idea of carrying out faithfully the instructions of the physician'.[17] Two responses to Pritchett's questions survive, but only one was apparently mailed. In the letter Nutting chose not to send, she defined the role of the nurse as something of a surrogate medical decision-maker.[18] Nutting was anxious not to appear self-serving and after deliberation she chose to respond by initiating a survey of physicians and public health officers, rather than superintendents of nursing, about the proper role and education of nurses. In the survey letter, potential respondents were asked to choose between two options. The nurse might be 'simply limited to carrying out as accurately and as skillfully as possible the order of the physician', or she might have a 'larger province in which she must be expected to use her judgment and act in some measure upon her own initiative'.[19] Regardless, both choices attest to the view that nurses themselves held: that they occupied, under direct guidance or more autonomously, a portion of the medical field.

Physicians and public health officers who were interested in the development of nursing also held widely divergent views about the nature of that development. What emerges from the extant responses to Nutting's survey is a sense that opinion ranged widely and that nursing was perceived as a divided occupation. Care of the sick was distinguishable from public health work. Leadership required different preparation than did daily practice. Gender determined role and had done so since time immemorial. In a revealing sentence, one physician summarized, 'Men discover what is new and bring it home, women make it useful, preserve and criticize it'.[20] What this same doctor called the 'psychical side of disease' was clearly within the woman's domain however, and the legitimate province of the nurse. In questions of emotional well-being, then, he stated, 'Women discover and men follow!' In the end, Nutting's survey achieved no clear-cut answer to Pritchett's question, and she was forced to admit that the profusion of professionals with views on the subject made it nearly impossible to achieve consensus.[21]

From the perspective of the late twentieth century, it might be argued that Nutting was actually attempting to negotiate a jurisdiction for nursing that would be acceptable to those who held sufficient influence to support or undermine it. During the second and third decades of this century a number of professions or aspiring professions approached philanthropists for support in establishing themselves through formation of professional associations, expansion of their work, and educational advancement. Occupational boundaries were especially malleable as new service-related professions gained in numbers and strength. Using philanthropic support to buttress a particular position seemed quite reasonable to strategists for professionalization. Those nurses closest to the policy-makers in the RF understood and employed this strategy, but they failed in their attempt, if indeed they ever intended, to fashion nursing as a profession independent of medical jurisdiction.

It was only natural for Rockefeller Foundation authorities and other professionals to see nursing as a subordinate field of work in light of the dominant voices of the medical and public health professions in the Foundation. Accepting temporarily Abbott's premise that delegation of tasks and not knowledge is characteristic of professions, these influential professional leaders would have had a distinct interest in controlling the work of nurses, while retaining ownership of the knowledge and technologies that were believed to underpin their work. The importance nurse educators themselves assigned to the inclusion of courses from other disciplines, taught by non-nurses, reinforced the perception that nursing had no separate territory. Without laying claim to a body of abstract knowledge, nursing fails one test of Abbott's definition of a profession. At the time, the impact of this lack of clarity was even more critical; nursing was unable to compete for patronage in the changing environment of Foundation priorities. It is insufficient to explain nursing's inability to obtain more funding by arguing that the occupation lacked the political, economic, or social power of some other professions, although it did. In the early part of this century nursing did not appear to offer the promise of generating new, abstract knowledge that other academic fields did.

The failure of influential nurses to clearly articulate the

boundaries of even practical nursing knowledge and work helped to spell the demise of RF attention. Mary Beard, who gradually assumed authority for nursing projects in America during Embree's tenure and beyond, often referred to the vast opportunities presented by nursing projects. But seldom did she specify in programmatic terms, the lingua franca of RF discussion, what precisely was to be achieved. Ultimately, the foundation of nursing, like that of social work and even of clinical medicine at the time, was practice-based knowledge. Anecdotal evidence, and even the statistical compilations preferred by many nurse reformers and their advocates, failed to be as persuasive to officials setting Foundation policy as the lure of basic science. As the RF redefined its mission from 'the well-being of mankind throughout the world' to the generation of new knowledge and dissemination of research findings, programmes geared mainly towards improving individual welfare were rapidly curtailed.[22]

COMPETITION VERSUS COOPERATION

Nurse leaders of the era seem not to have focused a great deal of attention on clarifying nursing's jurisdictional boundaries as they developed educational models within the university. Perhaps working out operational problems with hospitals, dispensaries and community agencies was sufficient trouble in itself. Even in the invitational meetings sponsored by the RF that created and underwrote the work of the Winslow-Goldmark Committee studying nursing work and education in America, leading nurses argued more about nursing's usefulness than its scope of practice. They made assumptions about what constituted nursing's legitimate field of work and took little apparent notice of the early incursions into the field by social work, teaching and psychology. Driven by a cooperative rather than a competitive model, nurse leaders stressed the inherent value of nursing and failed to limit the body of knowledge and the nature of work that nurses claimed. Without controlling the content of, as well as access to, nursing knowledge, and without limiting the work of its members and subordinate workers, nursing failed to meet the other criteria of Abbott's definition of a profession.

It seems that there were two pitfalls in tailoring nursing's reform agenda to coincide with the expectations of philanthropists, and nurse reformers fell into both. By focusing on the abuses of the hospital and the need for financially independent schools of nursing, American nurse leaders allowed RF officials to lose sight of areas that had become the autonomous work of nurses practising outside the hospital. By arguing over the classification and status of untrained personnel doing nursing work in settings other than hospitals, nurses failed to unite and exert control over a workforce. Whether nurse reformers did not recognize or simply chose to ignore the prospect of competition from emerging professions, they did not lay definitive claim to areas of *de facto* practice that were clearly outside the realm of medicine. Ironically, leaders continued to insist that nurses in public health receive some post-graduate training in psychology, sociology and education, indicating that they were aware of the distinctions between nursing and medical practice.

Competition and cooperation were then, as they are now, alternative strategies in cutting the social and health reform pie. Public health nursing developed rapidly between 1910 and 1925 as public health encroached upon the traditionally private realm of the domestic sphere. New fields of work kept appearing: industrial health, maternal–infant care, school health, rural care, mental hygiene, social hygiene, and social welfare, all were subsumed under the rubric of public health and so became the legitimate work of the public health nurse. However, advances in scientific knowledge did not translate directly into public information. As Ella Crandall, executive secretary of the National Organization for Public Health Nursing, pointed out, knowledge in the terminology of science did not 'greatly increase the popular intelligence regarding the prevention of disease'.[23] For public health officers managing limited budgets it was propitious for the scope of nursing to expand to meet the demand for new types of intervention. With appropriate generalist training, nurses might well be able to accomplish what would otherwise take two or three specialist workers to do.

Education and alleviation of the environmental causes of disease and social maladaptation featured as roles prescribed for public health nurses during the 1920s, functions that overlapped with the expanding roles of teachers and social workers. Teachers, social workers, physical education instructors and psychiatric workers were simultaneously vying for occupational recognition and attempted to define their own legitimate practice areas, or jurisdictions, as well. This put nurses and members of these occupations in direct competition for the same legitimate territory. One prominent public health nurse explained that social conditions presented barriers that prevented nurses from doing good health work with families.[24] Nurses needed to cooperate with teachers for very practical reasons. The nursing and public health literature of the era suggests that school nurses, overextended by heavy caseloads requiring in-home follow-up, agreed to provide health training for teachers in order to free nurses for home visitation. But alliances were not forged in all geographic regions or with all occupational groups competing for the same work.

In Nashville, Tennessee, occupational competition was illustrated in events that were partly subsidized by the RF during the reorganization of the Vanderbilt University School of Medicine. By the time the Rockefeller Foundation became actively involved in nursing education in Nashville, there were two competing agendas within the Foundation itself. One was to create a showcase for nursing education that would serve the southern states. The other was to aid the education of public health nurses to meet the needs for rural and community health care in the South. The effects on public health nursing and educational reform were particularly poignant in the context of the politics of philanthropy. Two schools with competing missions fuelled the internal debates at the RF. Bruce Payne, president of the George Peabody College for Teachers, viewed bodily failures as the root of southern social problems.[25] He had, therefore by 1917 attempted to establish a post-graduate programme to prepare public health nurses. Although it faltered during World War I, it was re-established in 1922.[26] Literally across the road, the Vanderbilt University School of Medicine was being reorganized and expanded, and a brand new hospital was built with RF funds.[27] The model for the enterprise was the Johns Hopkins Hospital, and a number of the medical faculty members were recruited from there.[28] A nurse training programme was essential for hospital operations, since paid graduate nurses were not yet used to staff hospital wards. Both Vanderbilt University and Peabody College applied to the RF for funds to achieve their separate goals.[29]

The applications precipitated a quasi-crisis within the Foundation. Ignoring the recommendations of the Winslow-Goldmark report that advocated financially independent and educationally sound programmes of nursing education, the interests of individual officers caused them to support one or another of the applicants. Embree was caught on the horns of a dilemma. Some wanted a hospital training school, others wanted to promote social and health reform. One policy was clear – the Foundation was interested in developing some institution in the South to prepare future leaders in health.[30] For almost everyone, the natural choice would have been to select Vanderbilt University, particularly in light of the educational 'experiment' of the Yale University School of Nursing, an outgrowth of the Winslow-Gold- mark report. However, the vision of those in control of the medical school and hospital was inconsistent with the educational agenda of nurse reformers like Goodrich and Nutting. On the other side was Beardsley Ruml, head of the Laura Spelman Rockefeller Memorial Fund, who wanted to expand the tra- ditional maternal–child welfare mission of the Memorial by sup- porting the development of social work.[31] Embree, too, was more sympathetic to the aims of Peabody College to develop a cadre of health and social reformers, some of whom would be nurses and others teachers and social workers. The question of who should educate nurses, at what level and under which discipline's jurisdiction, gradually escalated into a five-year-long debate both within the Foundation and among educators in Nashville.

Aside from personal agendas and institutional rivalries, there were genuine questions about whether nurses, teachers and social workers ought to be educated together, how they would divide the labour in actual practice, and who should decide issues of nursing curriculum. The authorities at Peabody operated with a vision of these occupations, and other 'new professionals' working together to achieve southern health. In the words of the director of the public health nursing programme, Abbie Roberts, the public health nurse was 'something of a social worker, a teacher and a person able to assume leadership in a community'. As such, she needed to 'touch shoulders with teachers, social workers, home demonstration agents, nutrition and physical education instructors', all of whom were educated at Peabody.[32]

The approach was inconsistent with the views of the most influential of Rockefeller officers and advisers, but touched a nerve in Ruml and Embree. Cooperation among the Foundation Boards had been difficult to achieve; to put together a programme that demonstrated how they could amplify the impact of phil- anthropy through joint efforts was a powerful incentive to these two men. Abbie Roberts's points about joint education and practical work between the emerging professions presented him with an opportunity to accomplish this and to develop an educational model for social work at Peabody College.[33]

Whether out of self-interest or genuine belief, the medical faculty at Vanderbilt opposed a joint venture. Social workers and nurses did not, the Dean of the School of Medicine argued, cooperate effectively in the South. Nurses could handle the bulk of the work if they had access to a highly educated social worker as a consultant.[34] Why did G. Canby Robinson, Dean of Vanderbilt's School of Medicine, take this position? One possibility is exactly what he told Ruml, that the chief of his department of hygiene held this view.[35] Waller S. Leathers was a physician with extensive experience in Rockefeller-sponsored public health activities in the American South. He had a clear idea of the scope of jurisdiction that might be had by a programme of public health that incorporated social aspects of illness and health. Leathers also saw public health nursing as falling directly within his own purview and was unwilling to cede any territory to Peabody College.

But there is another way in which Robinson's comment to Ruml might be construed. Was he suggesting that nurses were simply more effective agents of social reform, more versatile than social workers or teachers? Or did he mean that nurses were merely technicians, field workers, with physicians and social scientists generating the knowledge and methods by which they would labour? The correspondence between Vanderbilt authorities and their discussions with officers of the RF suggests that their perceptions of nursing tended to vacillate between the two.

In the end, the vision of cooperative efforts between the disciplines at Peabody College succumbed to aggressive competition from Vanderbilt University and to changes that occurred in the Foundation itself. Over the decade of the 1920s the Foundation had moved from support for educational experimentation to support for academic legitimacy. In this arena nursing was able to compete only marginally.

LIMITS OF MODELS IN NURSING HISTORY

Conceptual models that work under current conditions often fail to explain past events. Abbott's constructs of jurisdiction and legitimacy afford a perspective from which to view the waxing and waning interest in nursing's professional development on the part of the RF. Furthermore, the socio-political and economic environment did, in fact, limit nursing's professional development in ways that are consonant with the driving and constraining forces described in Abbott's model. The model is nonetheless insufficient to address certain other dimensions of the quest for professional jurisdiction, for example, the emergence of a caring profession from what was traditionally a domestic sphere. Similarly, the model may also fail to account for the development of other occupations that grew from women's work. Gender receives scant attention in Abbott's model, limiting its usefulness in historical or even contemporary applications to women's occupations. What was considered women's work may be an expression of the social milieu, but the nature of the occupational opportunities and the means women used to seize them need more detailed analysis.

Provocative questions remain about the choices made by American nurse reformers in their quest for professional parity with medicine and other more fully developed professions. Did nurses who had the attention of RF officers choose to ally more closely with Rockefeller medical men than with the emerging and predominantly female professions because of the inherent power of these persons or as a matter of occupational definition? Arrival at an historically accurate answer requires further study, but the choice, if not the rationale, was announced in the strategies nurse leaders selected to promote their agendas.

Alliances with powerful people in the Rockefeller sphere had proved successful in convening the meeting that established the Winslow-Goldmark Committee. Nevertheless, after working diligently to agree on a set of recommendations that would advance their causes, nurse leaders still chose a physician to present and critique the findings of the Winslow-Goldmark report, *Nursing and Nursing Education in the United States*.[36] It is true that this particular physician had been on the Committee and was historically a supporter of nursing's move into academia. But his views were not entirely consonant with those of the nurses who had served on the committee. Nurses most involved in the creation of the report seemed self-conscious about appearing to be self-serving. Male physicians and public health officers presumably were also perceived as having greater credibility in the eyes of industrial philanthropists and their managers than had women nurses, regardless of their social status. Nurse reformers consciously or unconsciously made decisions based on both power and gender – on what they believed was politically astute and socially acceptable.

Beyond these, there are other curious aspects that affected the drive for professional jurisdiction and academic legitimacy. The nurses who were most closely associated with the RF around 1915–25 firmly believed in the non-competitive model. They were politically and personally in opposition to those from whom they sought funding. While they were generally careful not to espouse views publicly that were too radical, they corresponded privately about cooperation and democratic socialism. Belonging to that generation caught up in social reform, their personal views may have extended to their professional actions. From all indications, other than distinguishing trained nurses from untrained ones, nurse leaders of the era refused to either defend nursing's jurisdiction from potential interlopers or to absorb them. Ironically, by allying with influential figures in medicine and public health, the small group of nurses who did for a time win a place at the RF table may also have inadvertently contributed to the Foundation's limited interest in nursing. The reorganization of medicine, the reformation of hospitals, and the restructuring of public health foreshadowed a declining interest in applied science in the Foundation. Organized philanthropy developed its own bureaucracy and the political environment shifted from progressive to conservative. Some of nursing's strongest allies were among those whose own spheres of interest were gradually curtailed, while a new generation of administrators supporting basic scientific research gradually took the reins of leadership in the Foundation.

The Foundation's waning interest in nursing should be understood not solely as evidence of occupational subordination to legitimate professions, but as a result of shifting priorities and power relations within the Foundation and in the social and political environment more generally. Nursing was, unfortunately, poorly positioned to withstand the withdrawal of RF support at this critical stage of development. The clients or public served by nurses lacked the power and possibly the desire to grant greater territory and legitimacy to nursing. Nurses themselves had not adequately defined nursing knowledge nor had they articulated the boundaries of their work. But while these conditions demonstrate the difficulty in establishing borders and holding them, particularly for women in the early twentieth century, neither necessarily relegates nursing to a subordinate 'settlement' within medicine.

The historical forces that impinged upon the search by nurse leaders for professional status and legitimacy were multiple. Abbott's model of occupational jurisdiction and control may be overly schematic in its representation of those forces. The lack of specific historical data relative to assumptions such as the knowledge-base of medicine during its developmental period in America suggests an acceptance of some prevailing assumptions about professional characteristics. Abbott's neglect of gender beliefs, personal irrational actions and random forces limits the explanatory power of the model especially for emerging professions. We need to continue re-examining the sociology of the health professions in ways that give full credence to the complexity of historical politics.

ACKNOWLEDGEMENTS

Portions of the research upon which this chapter was based were completed while the author was the American Nurses Foundation Teresa Christy Fund Scholar. The author wishes to thank the *Alpha Eta* Chapter of Sigma Theta Tau, and the Department of the History of Health Sciences at the University of California for additional support.

NOTES

1 See, for example, A.M. Carr-Saunders and P.A. Wilson, *The Professions*, London, Oxford University Press, 1933; G. Millerson, *The Qualifying Associations*, London, Routledge, 1964; and H.L. Wilensky, 'The professionalization of everyone?' *American Journal of Sociology*, 1964, vol. 70, pp. 137–58.

2 E. Friedson, *Profession of Medicine: A Study of the Sociology of Applied Knowledge*, Chicago, University of Chicago Press, 1970, 1988. The 1988 printing contains a new afterword arguing that the changing social and economic policies driving health care demand a new understanding of autonomy as an attribute of a profession.

3 A. Abbott, *The System of Professions: An Essay on the Division of Expert Labor*, Chicago, University of Chicago Press, 1988.

4 Ibid., p. 9.

5 Abbott, op. cit., p. 71.

6 Friedson, op. cit., p. 57.

7 Abbott, op. cit., p. 96.
8 Abbott, op. cit., p. 96.
9 1915–1955 Rockefeller Foundation Nursing Activities, October 1955. RF 1.1–100C–38–341, Rockefeller Archive Center, New York.
10 See R.F. Arnove (ed.), *Philanthropy and Cultural Imperialism: The Foundations at Home and Abroad*, Bloomington, Indiana University Press, 1982, especially, S. Slaughter and E.T. Silva, 'Looking backwards: how foundations formulated ideology in the progressive period', pp. 55–86, and E.R. Brown, 'Rockefeller medicine in China: professionalism and imperialism', pp 123–146; D. Fisher, 'The role of philanthropic foundations in the reproduction and production of hegemony', *Sociology*, 1983, vol. 17, pp. 206–33; M. Bulmer and D. Fisher, 'Debate', *Sociology*, 1984, vol. 18, pp. 573–87; B.D. Karl and S.N. Katz, 'Foundations and ruling class elites', *Daedalus*, 1987, Winter, pp. 1–40.
11 R.B. Fosdick, *The Story of the Rockefeller Foundation*, London, Odham's Press, 1952, p. 155.
12 Recommendations of the Conference on Nursing Education, 20 October 1925. RF 3.1–906–2–16, Rockefeller Archive Center.
13 Goodrich to Embree, 15 November 1928 and others. Records of the Dean, Yale School of Nursing, YRG 29A, ser. I, box 28, folder 309, Sterling Memorial Library, Yale University.
14 Embree to Crowell, 26 August 1925, 27 August 1925, and Embree to Vincent, 29 August 1925. RF 700C–19–139, Rockefeller Archive Center.
15 E.R. Embree, 'Adequate support of nursing education'. Notes for a speech made to the Central Council of Nursing Education, 15 February 1930, Embree Papers, HM 167, ser. III, box 6, folder 15, Sterling Memorial Library, Yale University.
16 Nutting to Pritchett, 10 June 1911, Nutting Papers, ser. 3, subser. II, fiche 1966, Mary Adelaide Nutting Historical Collection. See also, A. Flexner, *Medical Education in the United States and Canada*. Bulletin no. 4, 1910, New York, Carnegie Foundation for the Advancement of Teaching.
17 Pritchett to Nutting, 17 June 1911, Nutting Papers, ser. 3, subser. II, fiche 1966, Mary Adelaide Nutting Historical Collection.
18 Nutting to Pritchett, undated draft, circa June 1911, Nutting Papers, ser. 3, subser. II, fiche 1966, Mary Adelaide Nutting Historical Collection.
19 Form letter, Nutting to physicians and health officers, 15 March 1912, Nutting Papers, ser. 3, subser. II, fiche 1966, Mary Adelaide Nutting Historical Collection.
20 Cabot to Nutting, 22 March 1912, Nutting Papers, ser. 3, subser. II, fiche 1966, Mary Adelaide Nutting Historical Collection.
21 Nutting to Pritchett, 27 June 1911, Nutting Papers, ser. 3, subser. II, fiche 1966, Mary Adelaide Nutting Historical Collection.
22 E.R. Embree, 'Timid billions', *Harper's Magazine*, 1949, vol. 180, p. 28.
23 E.P. Crandall, 'The relation of public health nursing to the public

health campaign', *American Journal of Public Health*, 1915, vol. 5, p. 225.

24 K. Faville, 'Responsibility of the public health nurse for social phases of her work', *American Journal of Public Health*, 1930, vol. 20, pp. 165–70.

25 Payne to Embree, 1 May 1924. RF 1.1–200C–122–1512, Rockefeller Archive Center.

26 Tennessee Nurses Association, Public Health Nursing Section, *History of Public Health Nursing in Tennessee*, Nashville, TNA, 1960, p. 50.

27 Rockefeller Foundation History, 900–1–8–2126, Rockefeller Archive Center.

28 Ibid.

29 Payne to Embree, 1 May 1924, and Robinson to Embree, 3 May 1924. F 1.1–200C–122–1512, Rockefeller Archive Center.

30 Minutes of the Rockefeller Foundation, 21 May 1924.

31 Rockefeller Foundation History, 900–1–8–2150–51, Rockefeller Archive Center.

32 Roberts to Embree, 14 December 1924. RF 1.1–200C–122–1512, Rockefeller Archive Center.

33 Embree to Payne, 11 April 1924. RF 1.1–200C–122–1512, Rockefeller Archive Center.

34 Robinson to Ruml, 20 April 1925. RF 1.1–200C–122–1513, Rockefeller Archive Center.

35 Ibid.

36 Committee on Nursing Education, *Nursing and Nursing Education in the United States*, New York, Macmillan, 1923. See also, R.O. Beard, 'The report of the Rockefeller Foundation on nursing education: a review and critique', *American Journal of Nursing*, 1923, vol. 23, pp. 358–65.

Chapter 13

Children and state intervention: developing a coherent historical perspective

Jennifer Maxwell

INTRODUCTION

Within the social policy literature concerned with children and their families the definition and analysis of policy issues have been separated into two spheres: child care, and child health and welfare. The literature often appears to be more concerned with charting the history, and legitimating the occupational licence of the occupations working with children and their families, than with delineating the relationship between children and state action. The narrative of state action is obscured by the institutional and occupational segregation of policy implementation by different agencies and professional groups. Significant sections of the literature are best seen as part of the process of defining occupational jurisdiction and as an aspect of the professional image-making of the main occupational groups working with children and their families.

This chapter questions the validity of separating the issues into different spheres and argues that the dichotomy fails to present a coherent narrative of children and state action. Separating social policy for children into, on the one hand, child care, and on the other, child health and welfare, obscures the complex inter-relationships between children, their families, the state and various state agencies. Moreover, the traditional narrative fails to show the associated social regulation role shared between the two main statutory professions working with children and their families: social work and health visiting. The chapter concludes by suggesting the need for an alternative perspective which more adequately demonstrates the interconnections between social welfare agencies working with children and their families. Such a

perspective would endeavour to look beyond professional groupings in order to 'see the family as the focus of a network of
agencies which are in constant tension with each other'.[1]

CHILD CARE, AND CHILD HEALTH AND WELFARE

Modern social analysis has raised our awareness of the fact that
there is more than one way of telling a story; there is no single
narrative, no correct history. Historical accounts are interpretations of 'facts' influenced by the subjectivity of the writer and
the purposes for which the account is written. In the case of
children and state action there are at least two well-established
accounts that have informed social policy history and analysis.
These are: the socio-legal and the medico-social. Both have been
structured around the creation and development of the 'caring'
psychosocial welfare professions to address the social needs of
children and their families. The historiography of these developments has produced two perspectives on social policy which
reproduce the institutional and occupational segregation between
two areas concerned with children: child care, and child health
and welfare.

Two main areas of concern inform the socio-legal child care
narrative. The first examines legislative developments relating to
the use of state power to actively intervene and either acquire
parental rights or influence parental conduct where children are
believed to be victims, or potential victims, of family breakdown,
abuse or neglect.[2] The second focuses on the theoretical and
ideological perspectives informing the treatment of children in
the care of the state, and the policy statements and legislation
affecting parental rights and duties.[3]

The historiography of child care has been constructed around
the philanthropic and Poor Law antecedents of modern day social
service provision for children, the agencies and the professional
groups which have developed in response to and as part of the
socio-legal process represented by various Acts of Parliament.[4]
Social policy developments from the early 1800s are told as a
story of state and voluntary action directed at the 'social problem'
of particular groups of children: abandoned children, homeless
children, orphans, the children of the poor, and children classed
as destitute, vagrant, illegitimate, delinquent and criminal.

The history of child care is inextricably linked to the history of philanthropic initiatives such as ragged schools, Barnardo's children's homes and the National Society for the Prevention of Cruelty to Children (NSPCC). Statutory provision is related to the Poor Law services for pauper and destitute children. These included rudimentary residential care in workhouses, education and vocational training in workhouse schools, where boys learned a trade and girls developed skills appropriate for work as domestic servants, and the Poor Law system of boarding out children (the precursor to modern day fostering). Alongside the Poor Law, the literature also narrates the story of state action to address the problem of children labelled as delinquent or criminal. Reform schools and industrial schools are traced as the antecedents of the modern juvenile justice system.[5]

As the twentieth century progresses, perceptions begin to shift from children as problematic individuals to children as potential victims, vulnerable individuals, at risk of physical and psychological abuse or neglect. State action becomes more prominent, voluntary activity takes on a residual role, and social policy legislation and state agencies develop strategies to implement policies which sanction the surveillance of parenting and provision of alternative parental care.[6]

The main issues within the socio-legal child care perspective are identified as the rescue of problematic children and potentially 'normal' children from unsuitable environments, dysfunctional families and negligent or abusive parents. Intervention in family life is justified on the grounds of providing children with a socially appropriate upbringing and training in order that they become responsible adults. Within this framework social policy is identified and associated with the development of local authority social service departments and professional social work.

The socio-legal literature places child care prominently within the domain of social workers to the extent that certain social policies (for example, the 1908 Children Act, the 1932 Children and Young Persons Act and the 1948 Children Act) are analysed not as part of a wider social strategy but primarily as elements in the professional project of social work.[7] Acts of Parliament are examined in relation to changes in social work practice, theory and ideology alongside the administrative bureaucracy concerned with providing children with a 'normal' and appropriate childhood conducive to producing 'good' citizens.

The socio-legal framework of social work practice is clearly associated with legislation which sanctions state intervention in family life.[8] The historiography, however, embodies elements of the Whig model of social policy history. As described by Fraser, the Whig interpretation of history views developments in social policy as 'elements of progress on a path from intellectual darkness to enlightenment'.[9] Social policy developments are portrayed as the outcome of the work of heroic humanitarian reformers who inspire the wider society to a more caring, compassionate social conscience alongside a consensus for state-financed collectivist social provision for vulnerable members of society. The socio-legal child care perspective exhibits some of the characteristics of the Whig interpretation in its articulation of social policy for children as continuous progress along a linear path from rescuing children and providing care, to the modern-day concern with child protection. The concerns and emphasis of society might have shifted along the way but these are interpreted as increased awareness of children's social needs.

In contrast, the medico-social perspective has focused on policy issues concerned with the educational and physical health and welfare needs of children. The main issues of concern prompting past state action are identified as the need to reduce infant mortality and childhood morbidity.[10] In the medico-social arena we find a concern with state involvement and provision which places the emphasis on parental education, the development of good parenting skills in pursuit of optimum child health and wellbeing, and public health provision for children.[11]

Historically the medico-social perspective has been associated with the development of public health services for children. As with the child care perspective, child health and welfare also has its roots in the voluntary endeavours of the nineteenth and early twentieth century. The statutory development of child health and welfare services is linked to state concern about high levels of infant mortality, falling birth rates, especially among the middle classes, and the low level of working-class health. The fear of population decline and subsequent loss of industrial and military status to emerging industrial nations, alongside pressure group politics, prompted local and central government to provide health and welfare services.[12]

The emergent state bureaucracy of the period, sympathetic to the ideology of pressure groups such as the maternity and child welfare movement, incorporated voluntary activities into the developing public health departments managed by medical officers of health. Central and local authority public health officers and bureaucrats were important supporters of state-provided child health and welfare services. Public health pressure groups were dominated by members of the professional classes, especially by members of the medical profession, who used their status and work to influence and implement services at local level. Key administrators working at national level sympathetic to the aims of the pressure groups also used their position and resources to further the aims of the public health lobby. Szreter's analysis of the role of the General Register Office, established in 1832, demonstrates that this government department played a central and leading part in the development of public health provision throughout Britain during the Victorian and Edwardian periods.[13] Dingwall and Lloyd also show how voluntary health visiting was sponsored and reconstructed as a statutory social policy agency focused on infant health and welfare.[14,15]

The emphasis of the medico-social narrative shifts from services associated with the pre-school child to those provided for school-age children. The development of the health visiting service as the main agency providing for the pre-school child forms one strand of the narrative, and the provision of school meals and medical services forms a second.[16]

On the surface, legislation and policy which would traditionally be labelled as child health and welfare does not appear to be concerned with parental rights and duties. However, the underlying concern of both perspectives is the monitoring and regulation of parenting in order to ensure the appropriate socialization of children.[17] The medico-social perspective outlines the role of public health initiatives, voluntary endeavour and state education in influencing the social construction of organized maternal, and parental education practices and procedures. The underlying purpose of child health and welfare initiatives was to improve parental skills in order to facilitate better child-rearing practices to produce the same product as child care services: the 'good' citizen.

The construction of policies for children, as well as being divided into the two perspectives outlined above, is further fragmented and concealed within the histories of different interest and occupational groups. As noted by Cooter, children are encountered as actors in histories of: education; psychology; child employment; child protection legislation; in the literature on the late Victorian discovery of poverty; the rise of public health; the history of social policy; the origins of the welfare state and the growth of the caring professions notably health visiting and social work.[18]

To develop an understanding of the relationship between children and the state we have to unpick and select from these different histories. Given that children are secondary actors in these accounts, such accounts provide us with only fragmented pictures of the state–child interaction process. Interest group perceptions construct the issues into particularities of their own preoccupations which fail to address the complexities of the state–child interaction process, and become problematic when similar, if not the same, analytical tools are used to develop official interpretations of history.

Interpretations of the history of state intervention in the family contained within the child care and child health and welfare literature appear to be less concerned with delineating the relationship between children and state action and more interested in legitimating the occupational claims of social welfare occupations. The sub-text shows how different interest groups use similar, if not the same, analytical tools to develop official interpretations of history, interpretations which can and often are used to justify or make territorial claims for an occupation. I would contend that the traditional interpretations of children and state action provide the reader with insights into the legitimating and validation process of the main social welfare occupations which utilize the two perspectives in service of their own interests.

PROFESSIONAL JURISDICTION

Staking jurisdictional claim of occupational licence and mandate for a particular area of work is a fundamental prerequisite for any group seeking recognition as a profession. In the arena of work with children we find a number of occupational groups such as social workers, health visitors, teachers and child psychologists involved in the process of 'professionalization'. An important part of validating their territorial claims to the prestige title of profession involves asserting historical precedence within an area of expertise.[19] As part of the process of claim-making it is imperative for occupational groups to develop and promote their official histories to 'give their work, and consequently themselves, value in the eyes of each other and of outsiders'.[20] However, occupational rivalries, competition and conflict become an almost inevitable development, alongside the selective use of historical facts and analysis.

The literature on the occupations of social work and health visiting contains value judgements leading to historical interpretations which fail to show positive recognition of each occupation's contribution in the arena of child policy. Two recent publications, one on social work, by Parton, the other on health visiting, by Abbott and Sapsford, aptly demonstrate this.[21,22] Both publications ignore or fail to address the connection between child care and child health and welfare. Parton states that the aim of his book is:

> to provide an insight into three interelated themes: the nature of modern social work with children and families; the processes whereby elements of the social world become problematised and subject to social policy change; (and) the changes in the form of social regulation of the family in contemporary Britain.[23]

Abbott and Sapsford's chapter is concerned with the competing and contradictory discourses which inform health visiting practice and the resultant occupational and general confusion about the role and function of health visitors in social welfare provision. Both Parton's and Abbott and Sapsford's work are informed by Foucault's analysis of the relationship between medical and social science discourses, his exploration of the ways in which society has become increasingly disciplined, regulated and surveyed and the role that welfare state agents play in this process. Similarly, reference is also made to the work of Donzelot.[24] Donzelot draws conclusions about the working of modern welfare agencies such as social work and health visiting from his analysis of the relationship between the state, philanthropy and the family in nineteenth-century France. Donzelot's thesis suggests that nineteenth-century philanthropic organizations were utilized by the state as 'social policing' agents, intervening in the family on behalf of the state. It is from these philanthropic antecedents that welfare agencies such as social work and health visiting developed.

Donzelot's approach delineates a liberal state that fulfils a dual role as the non-interventionist guarantor of civil society and its interests, while at the same time intervening to regulate and influence the norms and values of its citizens. The liberal state is faced with a fundamental problem, in that the methods used to maintain social order must comply with the notion of a residual and non-centralized authority. This problem is overcome and resolved by a focus on socialization, especially the moral socialization of children within the family. However, fundamental liberal principles restrict the level of intervention which the state may overtly exert in the private domain of the family. This difficulty is circumvented by philanthropic endeavour which can legitimately pursue state objectives while maintaining a fiction of voluntary intervention in the family.[25] Donzelot describes three strategies used by philanthropic agencies to influence family conduct: moralization, normalization and tutelage or wardship.

Moralization is exemplified and documented in the work of the predecessor of modern day social work, the Charity Organisation Society (COS).[26] Moralization linked together poverty and moral failure. Financial and social assistance would only be given to families who could demonstrate that their own behaviour had not contributed to their distress. Families also had to show that they were willing to change unacceptable and antisocial behaviour identified by case workers. However, moralization is relatively inefficient as a preventive technique. It is a reactive strategy which can only influence those who are already identified as problematic citizens.

Normalization, the spread of particular forms of behaviour by educational instruction or example would appear to be a more effective strategy. The element of victim blaming inherent in moralization is reduced and external socio-economic factors are acknowledged as influential causative elements in personal social problems. Those in difficulties or individuals identified as potential problems to the maintenance of social order are confronted and attempts made to change their antisocial behaviour and develop, instead, socially approved norms and values. However, as a strategy, if agencies are denied observation of private conduct they can only react to behaviour which is presented by the family to the outside world. Normalization, like moralization, becomes a reactive strategy. To a certain degree modern social work practice approximates to a reactive form of normalization. Social workers are basically involved with clients who are already identified as having, or about to develop, 'social problems'. There is also an element of coercion in the social worker–client relationship, in that, as a result of being labelled as in need of social support, some clients may have been allocated social workers and forced into relationships they neither requested nor wanted.

In order for normalization to be most effective it is necessary for state agents to gain access to the private domain of the family and build influential relationships. These relationships should not be associated with negative labelling as a 'problem family', nor should they be identified with compulsion, and nor should they embody elements of legislative coercion. The third strategy identified by Donzelot, tutelage or wardship, takes on a proactive role and achieves admission into the private domain of the family. Tutelage is based on the model of teacher and pupil and is well demonstrated in the health visitor–client relationship, which allows the surveillance of the internal workings of families under the guise of social support. Private conduct can thus be policed and regulated without the use of direct coercion which might provoke resistance.

In reference to Donzelot's analysis Parton claims that, in respect of children, social workers are the successors to Donzelot's philanthropists. Parton states that: 'Philanthropy, and subsequently social work, developed at a midway point between individual initiative and the all-encompassing state'.[27] When it comes to laying claim to a philanthropic heritage with children, however, numerous commentators have documented the occupational claim of health visitors – a claim which historically may be more valid than that of social workers.[28]

Social work and health visiting both have their roots in nineteenth-century philanthropy. But the work of the social work pioneers, most notably the COS, was never specifically concerned with children. Their concern was the reformation of the adult character, the encouragement of thrift and socially acceptable behaviour. Any involvement with children was indirect through the relationship with the adult as parent. For health visiting, however, 'the focus of attention was the infant and child, the major target ... was the working-class mother'.[29]

When it comes to legislation we also find selective use and interpretations of the impact of different statutes. Fox Harding states that: 'The single dominating piece of legislation of the first twenty years of the century was the monumental 1908 Children Act'.[30] Parton also asserts that the 1908 Act symbolized the state's absorption of philanthropic activities.[31] According to this interpretation the 1908 Act sanctioned statutory intervention into the private domain of the family.

The 1908 Act consolidated numerous statutes dealing with the welfare of children. It reflected changing attitudes to the legal position of children and the responsibilities of parents and the state for children. But, as noted by Pinchbeck and Hewitt, the Act was primarily concerned with those children with whom the Poor Law was involved and its focus was the prevention of pauperism.[32] Dingwall, Eekelaar and Murray have also argued that legislators were probably less concerned with the physical deprivation of children than with their moral socialization.[33]

While Fox Harding and Parton's interpretations of the impact and importance of the 1908 Children Act might have some validity, they both fail to consider an equally significant piece of legislation, the 1907 Notification of Births Act. This Act had implications for significantly more children than those covered by the 1908 Act. The permissive 1907 Notification of Births Act, consolidated in 1915, created the conditions which made possible the access of health visitors into the private domestic sphere. Once in the home, health visitors were able to survey all occupants of 'a social category defined purely in demographic terms (initially home visiting to families with new-born babies, subsequently families with a child under five)... rather than predicted or perceived needs'.[34] The implementation of the Notification of Births Act overcame the problem of identifying, locating and gaining access to the family in order to survey parental conduct.

From these examples it is clear that, in order to comprehend the full implications of children and state action, it is necessary to develop an alternative viewpoint which takes us away from the divisions of child care and child health and welfare. Dingwall and Eekelaar consider English social policy for children during the nineteenth and early twentieth centuries and have argued that, as a starting point, the interrelationship between Donzelot's three strategies of social regulation should be considered.[35] Dingwall and Eekelaar argue that it is these which provide the environmental conditions for the growth, development and implementation of policies which have resulted in the various institutions and occupations constituted as primary agencies for the welfare of children. By addressing the relationships we can then attempt to analyse the connections between child care and child health and welfare policy.

In developing an understanding of the relationship between the family, children and the state, it is necessary to develop a concept which encompasses both the socio-legal and the medico-social. Instead of child care and child welfare our point of reference would become 'child policy'. A coherent analysis requires that we perceive child care and child health and welfare as merely different approaches to tackling the same concerns. The constitution of this site would be defined by the relationships of the various strategies of social regulation adopted by the state and its agencies. In the context outlined by Dingwall and Eekelaar social work and health visiting practice alongside the juvenile justice system, are interrelated. They are the outcome of strategies adopted to remedy and control two primary concerns: the inappropriate and poor child-rearing practices of some families and the need to protect the rights of children.

DELINEATING CHILD POLICY

The concerns of 'child policy' acknowledge that becoming a parent in the biological sense does not ensure that an adult can or will consistently maintain the standards of child rearing regarded by society as necessary and desirable. In cases that fail to approximate to social norms there is a presumption that the state should intervene between parents and their children. State intervention is defended by claiming a moral right to protect innocent children from various kinds of ill-treatment and inadequate or poor upbringing. Moral claims legitimate the state's use of extensive legal powers to overrule the rights of parents identified as inadequate, incapable or abusive. Intervention in the privacy of the family is also justified by the state's interest in children as future citizens. In this case the state has a duty to assist parents in fulfilling their parental role as agents of socialization and guardians of children on behalf of the state. As noted above, however, in liberal societies the state must not be seen to be too interventionist or coercive in the use of such powers.

How and when to use the coercive power of the state is therefore problematic. When should intervention take place? Who sets the standards by which families are judged? Should intervention be reactive, proactive or both? Most important, how is the state to know when poor quality child care is taking place and how are identification mechanisms to be applied to all the relevant population, that is, households with children? To overtly deploy state surveillance on such a scale would be unacceptable to civil liberty. Donzelot's thesis shows how such surveillance takes place through the work of state agencies interacting with children and their families.

Social workers are generally perceived as social police who intervene in the family on behalf of the state. Social work involvement and intervention in families may be initiated in a number of ways: individuals can present themselves as clients with problems or individuals are labelled as having problems and referred to social workers by other agencies. Social workers have a coercive role. They are identified with the authoritarian power of the state and their monitoring of families is publicly acknowledged. The surveillance role is sanctioned by statutory legal powers to intervene in families. The social work role is overt, in the sense that it is open to public scrutiny and observation. This is demonstrated by the level and tone of media comment and criticism of social work practice, especially in cases of child abuse.[36] It is very rare that health visitors are subjected to the same critical scrutiny, and significant that they seem to escape the same 'bad' press.

Traditional health visiting practice has been based on the systematic, routine home visiting of families with pre-school children in order to monitor their physical, emotional and psychological development. The continued practice of contacting parents of all newborn infants, and regular monitoring contained within 'routine' developmental assessments during the pre-school years, underline the fact that it is health visitors, not social workers, who have earlier and more frequent opportunities to make contact with and survey family conduct. Despite this, it is social work that is perceived by the public as a social policing agency.

Identification of health visitors with the social policing role is not fully acknowledged by practitioners and anecdotal evidence suggests that their client group do not perceive the occupation as part of the coercive state.[37] Health visitors believe that their role is significantly different to social workers. This perception may be related to a number of factors underpinning the way in which health visitors initiate contact and subsequently work with clients.

Despite attempts to develop health visiting as a family agency, health visitors commonly make contact with clients through the birth of a baby, a time, for most people, of celebration not crisis. Health visitors may visit families who develop 'problems' while they are part of their caseload. However, health visitors have not traditionally provided an interventionist service activated when things go wrong. Secondly, the philosophy of the health visitor as family friend and advisor serves to allow the invisible exercise of social control mechanisms.[38] It is their identification as a family friend which obscures the social policing function of health visitors and secures parental consent to the routine, unsolicited, visiting of families with pre-school children. But, as noted by Abbott and Sapsford, health visiting is very much an interventionist service with clear elements of social policing:

> Clearly, they [health visitors] have attempted to develop a non-judgemental style of work and to concentrate on developing good relationships with clients. They have none of the legal powers of social workers... nor any control over financial resources, nor do they have a legal right of entry into the home. The advice that they give does not have to be heeded, and there is little they can do to change the behaviour of individuals or families who resist their advice. Despite all this, they do attempt to shape the behaviour of individuals, to encourage them to conform to *societal norms*.[39]
>
> (emphasis added)

State intervention in families, articulated as social policy, takes different forms and covers different aspects of children's lives. Traditional commentaries and analyses of health visiting and social work have adhered to long-held ideas which reflect the incremental development of policies. By moving away from the fragmentation into child care and child health and welfare and looking instead at 'child policy' we can demonstrate the interrelated connections between different social policy and welfare developments. Contemporary developments in child protection illuminate clearly how inter-agency collaboration between social workers and health visitors is deployed in the surveillance of families.[40] As noted by Taylor and Tilley, health visitors collect confidential information on clients which 'they routinely pass on to multidisciplinary teams, including social services, probation and the police'. Health visitors play an important part in the surveillance of families but they hide their social policing role by 'going underground':

> In various ways the health visitor disguises her participation in child protection work. She does this both in terms of her public self-definition and in terms of patterns of everyday practice. Maintaining the requirement that a subpoena be served if she is to appear in court to give evidence sustains the public definition of the health visitor as one who unwillingly participates in the controlling aspects of child protection.
> The traditional medical ethic of confidentiality is propped up in the public demonstration of reluctance to disclose information passed on in private.[41]

By examining the strategies which underpin social policy for children and their families we can look beyond the occupational claims of interest groups. It then becomes possible to perceive the complexity of state intervention in the private domain of the family, and the interrelated nature of the network of agencies developed as part of the social welfare state. From this perspective the relationship between social work and health visiting is revealed. Each occupation represents a different strategy in the social regulation of families. To use a familiar maxim from the health and welfare field, health visiting provides a preventative service, social work a curative one, and the juvenile justice system acts as the agency of last resort for those who it is believed are beyond reason and change. Together these three strategies fulfil the needs of the liberal state to maintain moral order, without compromising the tenets of liberal society. Only when the interconnections between social welfare agencies are taken into consideration will we have meaningful analysis of the relationship between children and the state.

ACKNOWLEDGEMENTS

The ideas expressed in this chapter are drawn from work supported by an ESRC studentship. I also wish to thank Robert Dingwall, Julia Evetts and Anne Marie Rafferty for their helpful comments on drafts of this chapter.

NOTES

1 R. Dingwall and J.M. Ekelaar, 'Families and the State: An Historical Perspective on the Public Regulation of Private Conduct', *Law and Policy*, 1988, vol. 10, no. 4, pp 341–61.

2 G. Behlmer, *Child Abuse and Moral Reform in England, 1870–1908*, Stamford, Stamford University Press, 1982; H. Cunningham, *The Children of the Poor*, Oxford, Basil Blackwell, 1991; Dingwall and Eekelaar, op. cit.; L. Fox Harding, *Perspectives in Child Care Policy*, Harlow, Longman 1991; J. Packman, *The Child's Generation*, Oxford, Basil Blackwell, 1975.

3 Packman, op. cit.; N. Parton, *Governing the Family: Child Care, Child Protection and the State*, London, Macmillan, 1991; Fox Harding, op. cit.; J. Stroud, *Services for Children*, Oxford, Pergamon, 1973.

4 Dingwall and Eekelaar, op. cit.; I. Pinchbeck and M. Hewitt, *Children in English Society Vol. 2*, London, Routledge & Kegan Paul, 1973.

5 Packman, op. cit.; Pinchbeck and Hewitt, op. cit.; P. Seed, *The Expansion of Social Work*, London, Routledge & Kegan Paul, 1973; K. Woodroofe, *From Charity to Social Work*, London, Routledge & Kegan Paul, 1962.

6 Behlmer, op. cit.; Cunningham, op. cit.; Woodroofe, op. cit.

7 Packman, op. cit.; Woodroofe, op. cit.; Seed, op. cit.

8 R. Dingwall, J.M. Eekelaar and T. Murray, *The Protection of Children*, Oxford, Basil Blackwell, 1983.

9 D. Fraser, *The Evolution of the British Welfare State*, London, Macmillan, 1984, p. xxii.

10 D. Dwork, *War is Good for Babies and other Young Children: A History of the Infant Welfare Movement in England, 1898–1918*, London, Tavistock, 1987; B. Gilbert, *The Evolution of National Health Insurance in Great Britain*, London, Michael Joseph, 1966; G. McCleary, *The Maternity and Child Welfare Movement*, London, P.S. King & Son, 1935; G. McCleary, *The Development of British Maternity and Child Welfare Services*, London, N.A. M.C. W.C., 1945; A. Oakley, *The Captured Womb: a History of the Medical Care of Pregnant Women*, Oxford, Basil Blackwell, 1984.

11 R. Clarke-Crutchfield, 'Education for Motherhood at the Turn of the Century', *Health Visitor*, May 1987, vol. 60, pp. 151–3; C. Dyhouse, 'Working Class Mothers and Infant Mortality in England', in C. Webster (ed), *Biology, Medicine and Society 1840–1940*, 1981; F. Prochaska, 'A Mother's Country: Mothers Meetings and Family Welfare in Britain, 1850–1950', *History*, vol. 74, pp 379–99.

12 H. Hendrick, 'Child Labour, Medical Capital, and the School Health Service c1890–1930', in R. Cooter (ed.), *In the Name of the Child*, London, Routledge, 1992; R. Dingwall, 'Collectivism, Regionalism and Feminism: Health Visiting and British Social Policy 1850–1975', *Journal of Social Policy*, 1977, vol. 6, pp. 291–315.

13 S. Szreter, 'Introduction: The GRO and the Historians', *Social History of Medicine*, 1991a, vol. 4, no. 3, pp. 435–63; S. Szreter, 'The GRO

and the public health movement in Britain, 1837–1914', *Social History of Medicine*, 1991b, vol. 4, no. 3, pp 435–63.

14 Dingwall, op. cit.

15 P. Lloyd, 'The Management of Motherhood: A Case Study of Health Visiting to 1914', in A. While (ed.), *Research in Preventive Community Nursing Care*, Chichester, John Wiley & Sons, 1986.

16 Dingwall, op. cit.; Gilbert, op, cit.; Dwork, op. cit.

17 R. Dingwall, J.M. Eekelaar and T. Murray, 'Childhood as a Social Problem: A Survey of the History of Legal Regulation', *Journal of Law & Society*, 1984, vol. 11, no. 2, pp. 207–32.

18 R. Cooter, 'Introduction', in R. Cooter (ed.), *In the Name of the Child: Health and Welfare 1880–1940*, London, Routledge, 1992.

19 A. Abbott, *The System of Professions*, Chicago, Chicago University Press, 1988; E. Hughes, *The Sociological Eye: Selected Papers*, New Brunswick, Transaction Books, 1984.

20 Hughes, op. cit., p. 340.

21 Parton, op. cit.

22 P. Abbott and R. Sapsford, 'Health Visiting: Policing the Family?', in P. Abbott and C. Wallace (eds), *The Sociology of the Caring Professions*, Hampshire, Falmer Press, 1990.

23 Parton, op. cit., p. 3.

24 J. Donzelot, *The Policing of Families*, London, Hutchinson, 1980.

25 Dingwall and Eekelaar, op. cit.

26 Woodroofe, op. cit.

27 Parton, op. cit., p. 12.

28 J. Clarke, *A Family Visitor*, London, RCN, 1973; C. Davis, 'The Health Visitor as Mother's Friend: A Woman's Place in Public Health 1900–40', *Social History of Medicine*, vol. 1, no. 1, pp. 39–59; R. Dingwall, A.M. Rafferty and C. Webster, *An Introduction to the Social History of Nursing*, London, Routledge, 1988; Dingwall, op. cit., 1977; Lloyd, op. cit.

29 Abbott and Sapsford, op. cit., p. 135.

30 Fox Harding, op. cit., p. 87.

31 Parton, op. cit.

32 Pinchbeck and Hewitt, op. cit.

33 Dingwall, Eekelaar and Murray, op. cit.

34 Dingwall and Eekelaar, op. cit., p. 353.

35 Dingwall and Eekelaar op. cit.

36 M. Aldridge, *Making Social Work News*, London, Routledge, 1994.

37 S. Taylor and N. Tilley, 'Health Visitors and Child Protection: Conflict, Contradictions and Ethical Dilemmas', *Health Visitor*, 1989, vol 62, pp. 273–5; S. Taylor and N. Tilley, 'Ironing Out the Conflict', *Community Care*, 1992, no. 915, pp. 12–14.

38 Clarke, op. cit.; Davis, op. cit.

39 Abbott and Sapsford, op. cit. pp. 147–8.

40 Dingwall, Eekelaar and Murray, op. cit.; Taylor and Tilley, op. cit.

41 Taylor and Tilley, op. cit., 1989, p. 273.

Chapter 14

Women and the politics of career development: the case of nursing[1]

Ellen D. Baer

INTRODUCTION

The politics of career development, in one form or another, have probably shaped women's lives since the world began. In the last half of this twentieth century we have had the good fortune, and the parallel frustration, to participate in feminist debates and actions that have attempted to end, or at least ameliorate, the most negative career conditions for women. But as feminism has achieved certain success in gaining entry for some women to fields previously dominated by men, it has become evident that feminism has failed, thus far, to improve the continuing difficulties of the majority of women who still do what has long been called 'women's work'.

In this chapter, I present the particular case of nursing from the perspective of a nurse and citizen of the United States of America. I will argue that gender politics have hurt individual women who chose nursing as a career; that the same politics restricted the development of nursing as a profession and reduced its ability to contribute to health care as fully as it could, and still can. Further, I argue that, because nurses provide key personnel and services upon which the entire health care system depends, political attitudes that diminished nursing have had a negative impact on the whole system that all people – patients, potential patients and families, as well as professionals – must work to correct. Finally, I chastize modern feminists for not supporting nurses and nursing more vigorously, and conclude with some suggestions for societal responses that include feminist support for nursing.

THE CENTRAL FEMINIST DEBATE

A major dilemma for participants in the most recent feminist movement in the United States has been whether to advocate women's position as equal to or different from men's. Supporters of the 'equal' stance promote the entry of women into professional careers previously considered the prerogative mainly of men, and a few unusual women. Champions of the 'different' position focus on empowering traditionally feminine roles; though this latter group has been, in my opinion, much less vocal and successful than their counterparts in the 'equal' camp.

You may wonder, as I have, why both viewpoints cannot be sustained simultaneously. Why can we not support women's career choices no matter what they are, and use feminist forums to advocate women's right to choose what they will do with their minds as well as their bodies?

Wellesley College professor and women's historian Susan Reverby argues that the 'equal/difference' distinctions are rooted in people's differing consciousnesses and world views:

> Twentieth century American feminism has always struggled with how to make gender matter and not matter at the same time, how to value caring 'women's work' and how to demand that not all women be expected to do it. This tension ... is central to the dilemmas of modern feminism.[2]

The distinctions are made in the following way. To believe women are different from men means to adhere to the premise that certain womanly skills are inherently connected to femininity; that certain work is linked to female identity, rather than chosen as work; that certain characteristics are duties emerging from biological determinants and not rights that one chooses to exercise; and, finally, importantly, that women who choose traditionally female roles may not be choosing them at all, but may be, rather mindlessly it implies, staying within the boundaries of their female identity; perhaps happily and with contentment, but nonetheless, staying within that definition.

Conversely, the 'women as equal' group rejects the notion that there are characteristics or skills that are gender-connected. They believe that social characteristics are developed by acculturation, and that work is chosen in the context of that cultural perspective. UK sociologist Celia Davies' recent book gives an excellent review of these two positions and discusses the arguments of some of their proponents.[3]

Reverby has discussed the equal/different distinctions using 'caring' as a prism through which to examine them, because 'caring' is a particular feature of many traditional female roles. Reverby attempts to clarify the concern of the 'equal' group that it is 'difficult to speak about the importance of caring and connection without seeming to reject women's demands to be valued as individuals'.[4] This perspective suggests that individual autonomy is mutually exclusive of caring for other human beings; that, in caring, one loses his or her independent self. Consequently, the majority of people articulating support for feminism are wary of giving political support to women in caring roles, fearing that such endeavours work against overall feminist political goals. I do not agree with this fear or the premise on which it rests. First of all, the premise suggests that caring, and the intimacy involved in caring, costs something in autonomy; that to be connected means to lose your independence. I find this premise, on the face of it, illogical. In addition, it follows from this premise that professionals ought to have distant and mechanistic relationships with their clients. The implication is that allowing 'caring' to enter occupational enterprises subjects them to weakness.

Secondly, because of linguistic limitation and semantic overlap, the premise merges two separate spheres: the professional roles that involve care giving and caring, such as teaching, nursing and social work; and the personal roles of caring that engage parents, spouses and other family members of both sexes. Yet the nature of emotional attachment is entirely different between the two types of caring. Professional care givers are independent decision-makers, educated specialists who act in accordance with knowledge appropriate to their responsibilities, and whose autonomy of action is legally defined and has nothing to do with emotional closeness. They are not family members facing a poor report card or sick family member, caught up in situations for which they have no formal preparation or expertise.

I am a nurse, therefore my personal inclination as well as my feminist political position are oriented towards empowering traditional female roles like nursing, teaching and mothering. Further, as a teacher of nurses, I stress the professional obligation of nurses to maintain intelligent human connections with their patients – *not* to promote familial-like emotional attachment to those clients, but to create a humane environment in which people who are ill or needy in some way are supported to recover their health and independent status.

I believe that feminists who attempt to persuade women to abandon caring roles are in danger of demeaning the roles that women have traditionally occupied in society; roles that society needs and that many women and men enjoy filling. Additionally, I fear the societal outcome of encouraging distance, rather than caring, between people. As society moves further and further away from honouring women's roles, activities once primarily the focus of women's intelligence, interest and artistry are in decline and the quality of American social life is diminished by their loss. As the most talented women are drawn to approximate more and more to the life patterns of men, women's important traditions are in danger of extinction or relegation to the interpretation and practice of less gifted people, with serious, negative results for our social institutions.[5]

THE CASE OF NURSING

Nursing's difficulties with gender politics certainly existed from the beginnings of its modernization in the nineteenth century, and most emphatically were not caused by contemporary feminism. But recent feminism gave nurses hope that their problems would be addressed by a larger body of women who were gaining access to American boardrooms and media. Consequently, to many nurses, the main paradox, and disappointment, of contemporary feminism is that the 'women as equal' feminists have spent so much time and political capital gaining entry for women into fields previously considered men's domain, like medicine, that they have, perhaps inadvertently, demeaned fields considered women's province, like nursing.[6,7]

Feminist authors like Faludi rightly protest that the denigration of nursing, teaching, mothering and all care-taking fields was not instigated by feminists.[8] While this is true, the greater voice and success of the 'women as equal' feminist perspective has had the effect of seeming not to comprehend or support the values and ideas of people who *choose* society's care-taking roles. In fact, such feminists seem to refuse to believe that women who engage in 'women's work' chose it, thoughtfully and happily, with full consideration of other possibilities, and were not merely following their biological destiny.

Disconfirmation of care giving is not just aggravating to a few nurses who are tired of defending their intelligence. Because the health care system relies heavily on nursing expertise, the excellence and reliability of the whole system is threatened by this denigration of nursing. Members of all health professions, as well as recipients of care and their families, must assist in solving the problem. The decline in status of 'women's work' threatens the quality of life in American society in very fundamental ways. The ways that are particularly relevant for this chapter are those that affect patient care.

NURSING'S CENTRALITY TO HEALTH CARE

From the last quarter of the nineteenth century, when nursing moved from private homes to public spheres of activity, competent nurses have been the 'glue' that held the health care system together.[9] Historians indicate that reliance on nurses allowed hospitals to develop, families to trust the care of their members to people other than family, physicians to admit patients for medical interventions and surgeons to perform extensive operations, and all of them to go home at night, comfortable in the knowledge that a competent expert would be there to comfort the patient, interpret symptoms and signs, make valid judgements, and take appropriate action.[10,11,12] Those reliable experts were nurses, and without them, the work of health care and medicine would be greatly restricted. I emphasize competent, intelligent, professional nurses making informed and valid judgements, not barely-skilled ancillary workers who may recognize no pulse at all, but would not recognize a subtly changing pulse, an altered respiration, or lift the edge of a bandage to evaluate the nature and extent of ooze around a wound.[13]

One continuing societal misconception is that nursing is a sort of junior medicine, instead of being a discipline in its own right. Although there are, admittedly, many levels of nursing and kinds of nurse, professional nurses articulate a discipline of nursing in which researchers develop and practitioners apply nursing knowledge. The discipline defines nursing as doing for patients those things that patients would do for themselves if they had 'the strength, the will, and the knowledge that a nurse has'.[14] Nursing theorist Dorothea Orem has described the way in which, in practice, nurses substitute their knowledge and actions for the patient's when that patient is too sick, too old or young, or too infirm to care for him or herself.[15] The extent to which nurses substitute their judgement and actions for the patient's changes with the patient's condition. Some people need wholly compensatory care by nurses, others need only to be taught how to care for themselves.[16] Professional nurses decide which care is needed by which patients, set up the plan of care, assign the appropriate level of personnel to give that care, oversee, and evaluate it from beginning to end. Those activities require knowledge, judgement, and a whole array of practice skills that are based as much in the social and behavioural sciences as they are in the biological and medical sciences.[17] In summary, the central focus of nursing is the patient.

In contrast, the central focus of medicine is the diagnosis and treatment of disease. This disease perspective has dominated the development of America's health care system, even co-opting to its benefit many of the accomplishments of nursing, chemistry, biology and other basic sciences. What is less well understood is that nurses, in addition to providing nursing care, are involved with medical activities that contribute to diagnosing disease, and they also activate many of the therapeutic mechanisms that treat diseases. In fact, the success of disease treatment often depends upon the competence of the actions taken in the therapeutic process as much as it depends on making the right diagnosis and ordering the correct treatment. After all, what good is a brilliant diagnosis and treatment order if the person activating the treatment does not do it correctly, cannot interpret patient responses accurately, and does not have the judgement to intervene when needed?[18] Consequently, the success of medical practice depends, at least to some degree, on the competence and expertise of nursing practice and cannot afford a dilution of excellence in nursing.

Other health care disciplines also rely on nurses to supervise therapeutic regimes and manage health care environments in hospitals, homes and other agencies. In addition to initiating their own interventions, nurses participate in therapeutic plans directed by nutritionists, physical and respiratory therapists, social workers, psychologists, pharmacologists and the like. In fact, up until World War II, and even today over weekends and holidays, nurses, for the most part, manage those and other hospital departments when the particular specialists are off duty. Finally, hospitals, home care and other health facilities depend on nurses to manage patient care areas and supervise enormous numbers of ancillary personnel, in addition to providing patient care. Recent research by nursing professor Linda Aiken and her colleagues confirms these observations in finding that mortality rates among comparable patients are significantly lower in hospitals which are known for good nursing care.[19] In summary, it seems clear that the whole health care system depends on the intelligence, judgement, competence, reliability and problem-solving capability of nurses. The health care system cannot allow disregard for the importance of nursing to continue.

There is an assumption which abounds in the world (especially the television world) that the *only* thing nurses do is follow doctors' orders. Even if that were true, it would require an intelligent, well-educated, competent, responsible person to do the job well, and little recognition is given even to that limited view of nursing. Such is the 'disdain' for nursing that it is possible to render invisible the ideas, observations, knowledge, insight and experience of the largest group of health care professionals. The societal blindness to women's contributions that has had these effects on nursing is not only foolish and wasteful for society, it is ultimately enormously risky for patients for whom nurses are the closest connection and the most constant companions in the health care system.[20]

THE ROOTS OF THE PROBLEM

There are over two million nurses in the United States and women still comprise over 90 per cent of people graduating from basic nursing programmes in America.[21] Consequently, gender must be considered a significant variable in describing the roots of this disdain. It is not the only contributing factor however, because class and education are equal participants. But they also all go together, for who can say which is the chicken and which the egg? In the United States, women have only recently been afforded access to all the best educational institutions. It is working- and lower-middle-class women who have always needed to work to support themselves, and yet it is they who also have had fewer resources with which to purchase higher education.

Until World War II stimulated federal financial support for nursing education in the United States, nurses learned their craft in hospital schools where tuition was free because nurses bartered their labour as students for their education/training as nurses. By the time accreditation requirements and labour laws interfered with that arrangement, and academic schools of nursing opened in universities and colleges, the habit of thinking about nurses as 'workers' not professionals, trained in hospitals not educated in schools, was well established in America.[22,23]

Let me remind you of how nursing began as a formal system of paid work. Until the mid-nineteenth century, nursing care was given by women at home or in their villages. Men and untrained attendants, in most instances, provided what nursing there was in the military and in public institutions, where it was not considered 'proper' for respectable lay women to be. Religious orders like the Deaconesses in Germany and the Sisters of Charity in France had developed methods for religious sisters to care for the sick. But it remained for Florence Nightingale to secularize public nursing in England, and she began the system that spread throughout the world. Her idea was that respectable lay women would raise the level of care and bring to nursing the 'moral guardian' role of the Victorian woman, who had as her guide the 'four cardinal virtues of piety, purity, submissiveness, and domesticity'.[24]

But Victorian women could not work unchaperoned and retain their mantle of respectability, and reformers like Nightingale wanted very much for these nurses to be respectable in order to enhance the idea of reform. To describe her challenge in modern terms, Nightingale had to solve the paradox of gender roles in the Victorian era – respectable women could not work in hospitals, yet Nightingale believed that respectable women would solve the problems of care giving in institutions. The plan to admit lay women to a hospital nurse training school accomplished two goals simultaneously: it kept the women within the realm of respectability, yet made them available to do the 'coarse, repulsive, servile, noble work' of hospital nursing.[25] In a school, proper lay women could live in a 'Nurses Home', with rules of behaviour that included church attendance, strict discipline and study. Women with letters of reference from clergy and physician, acceptable breeding, and the ability to read and do sums were admitted to the school. But instead of attending classes as in a real school, the pupil-nurses or 'probationers' immediately went to work on the wards, providing all of the hands-on care to patients with the supervision of the matron. At the end of the period of study, initially one year at St Thomas's, the nurses graduated and were eligible for hire in private duty, district or visiting nursing.[26,27]

Following the lead of Nightingale, philanthropic, reform-minded women introduced nurse-training schools to hospitals in the United States in 1873. The American training schools also put their pupil-nurses to work on the wards immediately after entry to the school. Their two-year course of study, later three, provided some classwork, but usually it followed many hours of ward work and was only given to those pupils not still on duty. Notwithstanding the many injustices, the training schools were successful because they provided simultaneous answers to several American social needs:

1 Acceptable and meaningful work for single women seeking freedom and self-sufficiency in newly industrialized America;
2 'Protection' for women during their work in supervised enclaves called schools;
3 Respectable 'middling' class care takers for the sick;
4 Leaders from among the care takers who could be designated managers for the institutions in which the sick resided;
5 An inexpensive labour force to staff the hospitals rapidly proliferating by the turn of the twentieth century.[28]

The early strategies later became albatrosses. Nursing's early leaders persuaded a nineteenth-century audience of the righteousness of their cause through the use of women's reformist and inspirational rhetoric. By World War I, however, America's increasing love affair with westward expansion, science, technology and university education ensured that nursing, which represented none of these enterprises, remained in limbo, struggling for recognition. Nursing leaders from the earliest to most recent generations, such as activists Lavinia Dock and Dean Emerita Claire Fagin respectively, asserted their belief that the most fundamental cause of nursing's limbo was, and is, its gender-specific associations. The work itself has seemed infused with femaleness, regardless of the gender of the nurse. In consequence, historian Nancy Tomes pointed out: 'Women's professions have remained semi-professions because the prevailing views regarding women's proper sphere could not accord her an autonomy and expertise equal to a man's'.[29,30] For example, while the early nurse-training methods copied, to some degree, the apprenticeship models of education that simultaneously occurred in other professions like medicine and law, there were significant differences. Apprentices in medicine and law did not live in their workplace; were not held responsible for the practice of their profession prior to completing their training; and were not prevented from being married, having families, going home and maintaining other relationships during their training period. Pupil nurse/probationers' lives were so dominated by their training that their loyalties became co-opted by the work setting.

Until the Great Depression of the 1930s, few graduate nurses were hired by hospitals in America. All of the hospital nursing care was given by pupil-nurses; the training school *was* the nursing service department of the hospital. And, although this solution worked well for patients and solved the nursing care problems of the nineteenth century, it created for nursing a conflict between education and practice with which nursing has struggled ever since. Loyal to their past, nurses attached significance to the way students were taught, as apprentices, rather than to what they were taught. In allegiance to those traditions, many fought to maintain the hospital schools instead of accepting that university education would be a better way for the profession to develop. Modern-day criticism of nursing education is still aimed at where students should learn (in classrooms, laboratories and clinical settings), rather than at what they learn. And, in the proven manner of oppressed groups, nurses blame each other for nursing's problems, rather than the system.

Notwithstanding these difficulties, nursing flourished because it was one of the first jobs outside of the home that was considered acceptable for single women seeking independent lives during the years of tumultuous social change in the late nineteenth and early twentieth centuries in America. As people moved from rural to urban centres, and immigrants flooded into cities to join the American industrial revolution, they left behind familial and community networks that had tended them in ill health. In response to the resulting needs, the fledgling professions of medicine and nursing grew enormously. For women, nursing provided careers that made their lives full, earned them salaries, gave them a sense of their own competence, and allowed them to contribute to society in ways that would not otherwise have been possible.[31]

NURSING AND FEMINISM

Nursing presented a number of opportunities to American women of the nineteenth century. It offered them positions of power, running organizations, making decisions. Those attributes of nursing are no longer unique for women, and nursing must compete for recruits with all professions and industries. Many of these gains for women have been won by the feminist movement that began in the 1960s. Protest, litigation and hard-won legislation gained access for women to fields previously considered men's exclusive territory in the United States. However much I applaud these efforts, and think that nurses have much to learn from the political strategies of feminists, I am angry that feminists have *not* taken up the cause of the majority of women, who are still doing 'women's work'.[32]

It can be argued that to accomplish their ambitions in pre-feminist America, nurses and other successful women often maintained the facade of deference to men, in a sort of devil's bargain with social appearances. While seeming submissive, these women carved out for themselves powerful and significant careers without directly confronting the social primacy of men. Nurses like Lavinia Dock saw themselves as 'pioneer[s] in offering economic independence to women of education and good family whose only other alternative was "governessing", or needlework'.[33]

The women's movement of the 1960s, seeking direct, overt power, disdained the covert relationships constructed by women in previous eras and ridiculed those women as part of the problem the new women's movement sought to correct. Attacked by some of these feminists, and abandoned by former male supporters made angry by such feminists, women from older power networks, such as nurses, lost standing and position.

Too many feminists seem, ironically, to have bought the male model, and promote the 'masculine' professions as being better than the 'female' ones. I find that extraordinarily disappointing as well as hypocritical. Such feminists blame the victim, as it were: they blame the fact that women's professions are less powerful on the women's professions themselves and abandon them, instead of focusing their rhetoric and political clout on helping those groups to change their status.[34]

In the case of nursing, I believe that the basis for this devaluation rests on the assumption that they and others make that anyone free to make the choice would choose medicine, so that those who choose nursing must be lacking either the intellectual ability or the personal autonomy to aspire to medicine. Expanded, this kind of assumption holds true for other traditionally female careers as well, including staying home to raise children. The assumption is that all male-related things are better, and that anyone free to choose would choose the male option. One might well ask: what sort of feminism is that?[35] Personally, I do not know anyone in nursing who would rather be in medicine. Those I have known who have chosen nursing as a substitute for medicine did not last. There are differences in the practice and perspective of nurses and physicians that attract different people. Maybe a personal anecdote would help to demonstrate the differences.

In the early 1970s, when the nurse practitioner movement began, I spent a summer learning physical assessment at the Montefiore Medical Center in New York City. I was assigned to a surgery team and did many of their admission workups to practise my technique. Each morning the team met over coffee to plan the day, discuss who would do what procedures and the like. Then we went on early morning rounds to see our post-operative patients from the day before. The team would surge into the patients' rooms, do quick respiratory assessments and urine output checks, give the dressing a whirl, and off we would go to the next room. I found myself lagging further and further behind, because I wanted to stay with the patients. I wanted to work with them on their breathing, help them ambulate, do a good dressing change, answer their questions, explain things to them, and offer some personal comfort. I liked the intimacy of connecting with and relating to patients. I did not want to go to the operating room (OR), and when offered chances to participate in surgical procedures, I always said no – I found them boring. Finally the chief resident and I made a deal: I would whip through rounds with them and when they went off to the OR, I would return to our patients to give them nursing care. It was satisfying for me, beneficial for the surgical outcomes, and best for the patients. Why do people demean that?

What seems to be the case is that women's work, though needed, is not honoured in America; it is trivialized, even by some feminists. For example, instead of emphasizing the importance of the intellect and judgement required to care well for children or patients, American society emphasizes the menial parts of jobs, focusing on the diapers of mothers and the bedpans of nurses. Although every occupation and profession has its routine and trivial elements, its paper pushing and mind-numbing moments, those elements of women's work are made to seem primary. In consequence, many talented women feel embarrassed to acknowledge that they enjoy home-making, child or patient care, and are influenced to abandon such activities to paid substitutes. How ironic it is then to hear American politicians, scientists, media moguls, educators, and every other kind of pundit bemoan America's lost caring values.

Invented to soften the harsher realities of our society, nursing represents three persistent women's dilemmas: first, nurses are the prototypical women care takers in a society that undervalues care; second, nursing is an under-financed personal service in a nation that honours rational, entrepreneurial and product-oriented capitalism; and third, nurses occupy the down-side of America's gender-biased power structure. In consequence, I believe it has been too painful for women's studies scholars and feminists to look seriously at nurses' experience because nurses represent women's inherently unvalued place in American society. It has been easier to believe or hope that the job or salary or education or 'political incorrectness' of nurses was what made people uncomfortable with nursing. Most people simply do not comprehend how much nurses know, how important their work is, and how little they are credited.[36,37]

PROPOSED SOLUTION

All human beings crave respect for their knowledge, acknowledgement for their labours, and credit for their contributions. Lacking that in nursing in America, some nurses look elsewhere. They leave nursing for other fields or move into administrative, teaching, or quasi-medical roles where recognition is more easily gained. As a result, in the midst of huge medical advances and opportunity, nursing care is lacking, with the result that patients fear hospitals, families no longer rest easily, and physicians cannot get reliable care for their patients. In the United States, these factors have created a major, unacknowledged health care system problem, for recipients and providers of care. Further, I would argue that the newest American health care system problem, whereby institutions boost their profits by replacing nurses with minimally trained, cheaper substitutes, is an outcome of the same disdainful thinking which must be opposed by the same public outcry.

The outcry should come from feminists, recipients of care, their families, and members of all health care disciplines. Together they can employ some successful behaviour modification strategies to improve the image and position of nurses. These are methods that the American feminist movement has successfully used to make language gender-free in the United States; it has worked to force clubs, schools and professions to admit women; to control gender-biased content of textbooks and the public media, and to begin to garner equal pay for equal work. So why cannot feminists, patients, their families and physicians help nurses do the same thing for nursing?

Let us begin by not calling it 'medical care' as such any more, but health care – which includes all providers linguistically. Let us insist that nurses be admitted to the 'clubs' of health care and gain representation on the boards of hospitals and agencies and government committees where the policies are set and the big decisions made. Let us erase militaristic words like 'orders' and create a vocabulary which focuses on the patient and on care, such as 'patient treatment plans' instead of 'doctor's orders'. Let us allow certain nursing specialists to write their nursing treatment plans in the same book in which all providers except nurses currently write their treatment plans. Let us secure for nurses financial arrangements that are not only equitable in salary with other professionals, but which also ensure that insurance reimbursement for nurses' work goes directly to nursing and the nurses who earned the reimbursement, rather than into the hospital's general accounts which do not credit nursing. Crediting to nursing the income that nurses earn for the institution would make nursing obvious as the revenue-producing centre that it is, rather than the cost centre it is always seen as by accountants and business people in hospital offices who seem to make the health care decisions these days, yet have little direct knowledge about or involvement in patient care. And let us challenge the attitudes of people who say to young nurses: you're too smart to be a nurse. *All* people *must* realize that, eventually, *everyone* is glad to have a smart nurse taking care of them or their family members.[38]

CONCLUSION

Nurses are the prototypically invisible women whose minds, hearts and hands have shaped a huge industry, yet who are ignored equally by traditionally male power brokers and new feminist status builders. American society is now moving further and further away from honouring women's roles, with the encouragement and assistance of feminists who argue that talented women, as equals to men, should do what men do. They seem not to have considered that women can be equal to men and do what women do. The solution for women and for society is to make women's roles as attractive and remunerative as men's, so that talented people are drawn to fulfil all dimensions of human existence.

In the opening paragraphs, I discussed the philosophical distinctions feminists draw between women as 'equal to' and 'different from' men. I would like to conclude by saying that I reject those distinctions. I find it ludicrous to discuss women's work, women's contributions and women's sphere by comparing it to men's. I am mystified by the logic of people who call themselves 'feminists' using terms like 'women as equal to' or 'different from' men, as if being a man were the essential bedrock on which human endeavors were based. Further, as Davies argues: 'Ignoring difference, acting as equal is often an important strategy for women and at an individual level is sometimes a spectacularly successful one. But it leaves patriarchal cultures 'intact.'[39] Finally, I strongly believe that any group calling itself 'feminist' is obligated to lobby on behalf of all women, not just those who occupy what seems to them to be the more 'politically correct' end of the human continuum. Any other position makes feminists part of the problem, not part of the solution for women.

In closing, I would like to share with the reader a wonderful and relevant quote from Ethel Manson Fenwick, who was an organizer of the British Nurses Association in 1887, editor of the *Nursing Record* later to become the *British Journal of Nursing*, and a strong antagonist of her contemporary Florence Nightingale regarding the state registration of nurses. Fenwick aptly summed up the situation when she said in 1887: 'The Nurse question is the Woman question, pure and simple. We have to run the gauntlet of those historic rotten eggs.'[40]

NOTES

1 This chapter began with an article published in the *New York Times* in 1991. Later that year, I expanded the essay to present in a panel discussion at the University of Virginia Health Sciences Centre, the proceedings of which were published in 1994. The paper was further developed for the conference 'Nursing, Women's History and the Politics of Welfare', at the University of Nottingham, England. At that time, I incorporated ideas that had been published earlier in various chapters and articles. I have tried to guide the reader to those earlier materials through the accompanying citations.

2 S.-M. Reverby, ' "Even her Nursing Friends see her as 'only' a Feminist" . . . and Other Tales of the Nursing–Feminism Connection', *Nursing and Health Care*, 1993, vol. 14, no. 6, pp. 298–9.

3 C. Davies, *Gender and the Professional Predicament in Nursing*, Milton Keynes/Philadelphia: Open University Press, 1995, pp. 19–42.

4 Reverby, op. cit., p. 300.

5 E.D. Baer, 'Nurses', in R. Appel (ed.), *Women, Health and Medicine in America: A Historical Handbook*, New York: Garland, 1990, pp. 459–75.

6 E.D. Baer, 'The Feminist Disdain for Nursing', *New York Times*, Op. Ed., 23 February 1991, A25.

7 E.D. Baer, B. Brodie, J.C. Kirchgessner and E.W. Hook, 'Is there a Feminist Disdain for Nursing?', *The Pharos of Alpha Omega Alpha*, 1994, vol. 57, no. 3, Summer, pp. 36–40.

8 S. Faludi, *Backlash: The Undeclared War against American Women*, New York: Crown, 1991.

9 L. Thomas, *The Youngest Science: Notes of a Medicine Watcher*, New York: Viking Press, 1983, p. 67.

10 C.E. Rosenberg, *The Care of Strangers, the Rise of America's Hospital System*, New York: Basic Books, 1987, pp. 8–9.

11 S.M. Reverby, *Ordered to Care: The Dilemma of American Nursing*, New York: Cambridge University Press, 1987.

12 G.D. Stewart, 'Graduation Address', *St Vincent's Leaves*, Newsletter of the St Vincent's Hospital Training School for Nurses, New York: Sisters of Charity Archives at the College of Mt St Vincent, 1905, p. 8.

13 Baer *et al.*, 1994, op. cit., p. 36.

14 V. Henderson in *Nursing in America: A History of Social Reform*, A Video Documentary, New York: National League for Nursing, 1990.

15 D. Orem, *Nursing: Concepts of Practice*, 4th edn, St Louis: Mosby Yearbook.

16 J. Fawcett, *Analysis and Evaluation of Conceptual Models of Nursing,* Philadelphia: F.A. Davis, 1983, p. 186.
17 Baer *et al.*, op. cit., p. 36.
18 Baer *et al.*, op. cit., pp. 36–7.
19 L.H. Aiken, H.L. Smith and E.T. Lake, 'Lower Medicare Mortality among a Set of Hospitals known for Good Nursing Care', *Medical Care*, 1994, vol. 32, no. 8, pp. 771–87.
20 Baer *et al.*, op. cit., p. 37.
21 *Nursing Data Review 1994*, New York: National League for Nursing, 1994, p. 76.
22 E.D. Baer, 'American Nursing: 100 Years of Conflicting Ideas and Ideals', *Journal of the New York State Nurses' Association*, 1992, vol. 23, no. 3, pp. 16–21.
23 Baer *et al.*, op. cit., p. 37
24 B. Welter, 'The Cult of True Womanhood 1820–1860', *American Quarterly*, 1966, vol. 18, Summer, p. 152.
25 Nightingale quoted in M. Baly, *Florence Nightingale and the Nursing Legacy*, London: Croom Helm, 1986, p. 21.
26 Baer, 1992, op. cit., p. 20.
27 Baer *et al.*, op. cit., p. 37.
28 Baer, 1990, op. cit., p. 461.
29 N. Tomes, 'Nursing Historiography Review Essay', unpublished manuscript, Philadelphia: University of Pennsylvania, undated, p. 6.
30 Baer, 1990, op. cit., p. 465.
31 Baer, 1992, op. cit., p. 20.
32 Baer, 1991, op. cit., A25.
33 L.L. Dock and I.M. Stewart, *A Short History of Nursing*, 2nd edn, New York: G.P. Putnam, 1925, pp. 9–10.
34 Baer *et al.*, op. cit., p. 38.
35 Baer *et al.*, op. cit., p. 38.
36 Baer, 1990, op. cit., pp. 474–5.
37 Baer, 1991, op. cit., A25.
38 Baer *et al.*, op. cit., pp. 38–9.
39 Davies, op. cit., p. 37.
40 Fenwick quoted in L.L. Dock, *A History of Nursing*, Vol III, New York: G.P. Putnam, 1912, p. 33.

Chapter 15

Nurses in the archives: archival sources for nursing history

Lesley A. Hall

Nursing tends to be less well-documented than medicine. As discussed later in this chapter, this has a good deal to do with assumptions about its nature. For centuries it tended to be regarded as one aspect of the normal womanly role, and even if a degree of learned skill might be conceded, the learning would largely have taken place orally and by informal apprenticeship experience. It involved physical, hands-on competence rather than qualifications associated with formal learning and scholarship.

Sources through which the history of nursing could be traced were described by Foster and Sheppard in *Rewriting Nursing History* in 1980.[1] Since then, increasing interest in the subject has led to the unearthing of additional materials, while the availability of hitherto unused archives has also stimulated research. It is therefore worth describing the state of affairs some fifteen years on from then.

This chapter falls into four parts: a general description of what archives are and are not; what kind of information about nurses can be found in various kinds of archival sources; hospital records and how to find them; and wider questions of the preservation of archives. A list of useful addresses is appended. Works cited in footnotes provide recommended further reading.

WHAT ARCHIVES ARE AND WHAT THEY ARE NOT

Archives were not created with the historian in mind; they originate as records of transactions deemed of sufficient significance to be written down. Things of that importance usually involve, though not exclusively, at some level, a financial transaction. However, in societies of increasing literacy, more and more things of less and less importance are recorded. This is not necessarily such an advantage for the historian as it sounds, as without proper programmes of control, vast amounts of ephemeral or duplicate material may be being kept. The sight of storerooms full of vast quantities of paper of no further current relevance has sometimes led to the wholesale disposal of archives in the name of efficiency, the important along with the trivial.

Some items which are popularly described as 'archives' are not technically speaking archives at all. Photographs may be part of an archive – for example, if they relate to the activities of a particular institution – but a collection of photographs is not in itself an archive. While the journal of an organization is not normally an archive, a set retained for editorial reference purposes by the organization itself is. A set of scrapbooks or files of press-cuttings about an institution or organization or the field in which it is interested is archival, but stray scrapbooks or collections of cuttings are not. Archives are, as it were, a by-product, they were not self-consciously created for their own sake.

LOOKING FOR NURSES IN THE ARCHIVES

Foster and Sheppard pointed out that there are few or no records of nursing as such before the great nineteenth-century professionalization of nursing and its reform into a self-conscious profession.[2] However, there are oblique ways of approaching the history of nursing before this period. Records of hospitals do survive from the Middle Ages, though 'hospital' had a somewhat different meaning then, and few cared for the non-leprous sick poor. Surviving records might include charters of foundation, bequests, account books recording payments, legal records and the accounts of investigations in cases of suspected malfeasance. These supply very little information about the kind of nursing care, if any, that was provided, although apparently the sick received bed rest, warmth, cleanliness and a diet probably more adequate than they would have had outside. Clothing was sometimes also provided to replace infested garments. The sisters responsible for nursing care might be inspected to see how well they supervised and visited the sick, and how they ministered to them and fed them, but this is about as far as details of nursing practice go. What is not in records is sometimes as revealing as what is, since the assumptions behind omissions, for example, that everyone knows what is involved in attendance upon the sick, can be illuminating.

Such assumptions constitute a major problem in dealing with nursing in the pre-professionalization era. Much nursing care must have simply consisted in doing for patients things they were too infirm to do for themselves, including washing and feeding them, and this kind of attendance upon the sick would largely have taken place within the home and devolved upon female family members, and thus was not the sort of activity which would be routinely documented. The association of nursing with the standard female gender role was acknowledged by Florence Nightingale in her *Notes on Nursing*, addressed to those caring for the sick within their own homes, in which she indicated that 'every woman must, at some time in her life, become a nurse'.[3] Nursing sick members of the family was an extension of the general female responsibility for questions of domestic hygiene. There would seem to have been a certain amount of philanthropic voluntarism in the field of the care of the sick, not merely on the level of 'Lady Bountiful' dosing her tenants but of mutual aid between women in local communities; this kind of thing is highly unlikely to show up in archival sources, as much of it took place among the illiterate or barely literate.

However, especially in higher social classes, nurses were sometimes hired to care for members of the family, something that can be traced in account books, and possibly stray comments in family correspondence and diaries. Again, there is unlikely to be much record of what they actually did for their patients. They might have had some hospital experience in the care of the sick – perhaps the most famous fictional case is Grace Poole in *Jane Eyre*, who seems to have had prior experience of attendance upon the insane before being hired by Mr Rochester to look after the first Mrs Rochester.

It seems probable that hospital nurses in the eighteenth and early nineteenth centuries had some sort of training, even if it was only a combination of prior experience of tending the sick in their own family, an informal apprenticeship of induction into the customs of a particular hospital and the idiosyncrasies of the various doctors, and the accumulation of further hands-on experience. Nurses were drawn from the same class as domestic servants and much of their work was at that level: many of the tasks later deemed to be the purlieu of the professional nurse were undertaken by the doctor or surgeon and his pupils and 'dressers', as this term suggests. In some hospitals the less bedridden patients were expected to assist in nursing care under the supervision of the nurses.

However, a cadre of experienced nurses seems to have existed only in voluntary hospitals. The system under the Poor Law was for the haler female paupers to take care of the sick. In some cases before the 1834 New Poor Law, nurses were occasionally sent out at parish expense to attend the sick poor in their own homes, and this is something that can be traced in archives since such nurses were paid by the parish.[4] There is, however, at least one instance of a workhouse inmate being sent out for home nursing attendance duties in return simply for her keep within the workhouse.[5] (One hopes this nurse perhaps got some kind of privilege, such as better diet, though it might well have been an increased drink allowance.)

Because of the often informal nature of nursing care, and assumptions about the kind of care it was, there is thus relatively little to be gleaned about its practice from archival sources, though prescriptive literature, such as manuals of domestic hygiene, may include chapters on the care of the sick, and hospital regulations may indicate what nurses' duties were supposed to be. Archives may reveal indicators of status such as how much nurses were paid, and their conditions of service: hospital minutes may also record complaints against them, though not necessarily for defects in nursing, as in the case of the nurse at the Radcliffe Infirmary, Oxford, reproved for letting a patient put his arm around her.[6]

The records of nursing began to proliferate in the nineteenth century, though informal nursing within the community would have continued unrecorded, while at higher social levels nursing engaged in on a voluntary and philanthropic basis would not necessarily be recorded in any institutional archives. Towards the end of her life the Quaker philanthropist and reformer Elizabeth Fry was involved in establishing a Protestant Nursing Sisterhood, to nurse the sick poor in their own homes (and sometimes the better-off for a fee). The minutes of this body survive embedded within the Queen's Nursing Institute archives, also one register of nurses. The hazards which face historical material are nicely illustrated by a note inside the front cover, dated December 1941, which reads:

It was decided by the Committee, that this ledger, the first in use at the Institution, be preserved, and that all others of later date, be sent to the local Waste Paper Salvage Committee in response to the urgent appeal for waste paper required in the making of munitions.[7]

This is a classic instance of why so many gaps exist in the historical record.

The lady philanthropists of the Committee did not themselves engage in nursing work. Those wishing to become Protestant Nursing Sisters applied to the Committee with testimonials from a clergyman or minister, a lady or a respectable housekeeper: once accepted as Probationers, they were sent for hospital training at either the London Hospital or Guy's – and in at least one early case, to Hanwell Asylum for experience in nursing the insane. This training appears to have taken only a few months: the first nurse in the register went to the London in August and was sent out on her first case in October. Reports were submitted on the nurses. This first nurse was not only 'tender in the management of her surgical duties' but 'very soothing' to her patient's mind 'on religious subjects in her judicious choices from scripture'.[8]

This was one of a number of nursing organizations which aimed to provide home nursing care. There was a strong relationship between such endeavours and religious enthusiasm. An inspiration was the Protestant Institute of Deaconesses at Kaiserwerth, and the 'Oxford Movement' with its associated revival of 'High' ritualistic practices within the Anglican Church which encouraged the development of nursing sisterhoods such as the Park Village Community established in 1845 under the aegis of Pusey (a leading figure in this movement), and Priscilla Seddon's Sisters of Mercy formed in 1848. St John's House was set up in 1848 to train nurses under the supervision of a clergyman, and King's College Hospital began receiving pupil nurses of higher social class from 1856, developments for which archival sources still survive.[9] These initiatives serve to undermine the still-popular mythology that nursing in the nineteenth century was in the hands of gin-sodden Sarah Gamps until Florence Nightingale undertook its reform. Nightingale herself was more of an administrator and a reformer than a hands-on practitioner of nursing but her ideas

were influential if only because they articulated, in the mouth of
a national heroine, changing perceptions of the role of the nurse.

With increasing emphasis on the need to train nurses, and the
enforcement of standards of nursing care within hospitals, nursing
becomes more visible in archive sources, though largely in the
more advanced voluntary hospitals. These tend to present a probably untypical view of nursing at the period. There were conflicts
between nurses of this new school, owing allegiance to a matron
of their own sex and forming a separate hierarchy of their own
within a hospital, with a very definite vision of what nursing was
about, and doctors and administrators who still saw nurses as
glorified domestic servants and handmaidens to themselves.
Judith Moore has documented in detail the struggles within King's
College and Guy's Hospital, involving St John's House Sisterhood.[10] The records which may survive to illuminate changes
within hospital nursing will include the general administrative
minutes, possibly separate nursing committee minutes, matrons'
reports, and registers of nurses, as well as training records and
reports. The survival of such records has been, like that of most
archives, haphazard. Hospital records are discussed more fully
below.

However, not all nursing took place in hospitals, and with the
increasing professionalization of home nursing provision this is
also increasingly reflected in archival sources. Elizabeth Fry's
Protestant Nursing Sisters have been mentioned; reference perhaps ought also to be made to the Ranyard Bible Nurses who,
like the Fry nurse mentioned above, gave spiritual consolation as
well as nursing care. In fact their initial function was more
religious than medical, although they gave assistance in matters
of domestic hygiene which perhaps makes them precursors of
health visitors. In the 1860s Mrs Ranyard was able to initiate
training of poor women as itinerant nurses for the slums. As with
Fry's Protestant Nursing Sisters, their training took place in Guy's
Hospital. Their records survive in the Greater London Record
Office. The records of the Queen's Nursing Institute (QNI), chartered 1889, are now in the Contemporary Medical Archives
Centre (CMAC) and cataloguing is in progress (August 1996).
Nearly 600 items (apparently a selection from a previous larger
series) relating to the affiliation of local nursing associations to
the QNI and their regular inspection, 1890–1948, were transferred
to the Public Record Office (class PRO 30/63). Records of several

hundred district nursing associations survive in local record offices, according to the CMAC register of sources held in other repositories; this does not include cases where local authorities contracted for district nursing services.

However, there are still considerable problems involved in pursuing nurses through archival sources. The 'Note on Sources' in Summers' *Angels and Citizens* illuminates these and reveals how important a general knowledge of the period is to the pursuit of relevant archival material.[11] She remarks, specifically in the context of military nursing, that 'Official sources are very disappointing'. War Office records contain scanty material on female nurses, although there is evidence that some files were destroyed, and some others recorded in 1931 have disappeared. However, other classes of War Office material relating to hospital administration, etc. shed some light on the position of female nurses within it. The nineteenth-century practice of senior officials taking documentation away with them on retirement means that official records can be scant, although sometimes stray documents turn up in less official collections, such as among the Muniment Collection of the Royal Army Medical Corps (now in the CMAC at the Wellcome Institute) – although nursing is not one of the strengths of this collection. The archives of voluntary agencies can supplement official records, if they survive, and so can papers of private individuals. For example, Summers points out that Elizabeth Haldane was the sister of the Secretary of State for War, sat on the Territorial Field Nursing Service Nursing Board, and was the 'confidante' of both the Director-General of Army Medical Services and the Matron in Chief of Queen Alexandra's Imperial Military Nursing Service, which provided her with a combination of formal and informal contacts with both official and voluntary agencies. However, although records are there and available to those who dig for them, as Summers remarks, they seldom enable us 'to hear the voices of the nurses themselves'.

The mirror-image of archives widely dispersed throughout diverse collections is that of archives which become embedded in those of another body or person. In some cases, predecessor bodies' archives are to be found among those of their successors, as are those of associated organizations. Among the records of the Queen's Nursing Institute there are to be found the surviving records of Elizabeth Fry's Institution of Protestant Nursing Sisters and of a number of local Nursing Associations in the

Metropolitan area; and records of the William Rathbone Staff College. A perhaps analogous case is the situation in which a wife's papers are embedded among or enmeshed with her husband's. In the CMAC, nurse training notebooks of Ada Sowerby during the 1920s form a clearly distinct group among the papers of her husband, the radiologist F.G. Spear, while within the papers of Sir Albert and Lady (Katherine) Cook about their work in Uganda as medical missionary and missionary nurse, Lady Cook's papers are less distinct as a group because of their common interests. A similar situation pertains in the archives of the Royal College of Nursing (now held in Edinburgh), which include the records of a number of other bodies, which have been described by the Royal College of Nursing archivist, Susan McGann.[12]

There are some nursing records in the Public Record Office: archives of the General Nursing Council, 1919–83 (records of the English National Board for Nursing, Midwifery and Health Visiting will be transferred under the thirty-year rule), Joint Board for Clinical Nursing Studies, 1966–83, and some Queen's Nursing Institute records as mentioned above, as well as items relating to national nursing policy in various administrative classes.

One area for which records of nursing do survive in considerable quantity is war, although Anne Summers has demonstrated some of the problems in locating and retrieving them, at least in the pre-World War I period. However, the British Red Cross holds archives including records of the Voluntary Aid Detachment, the Imperial War Museum has quantities of documents (see the return compiled for the Wellcome Institute Medical Archives and Manuscripts Survey, available in the Wellcome Institute Library), and the Queen Alexandra's Royal Army Nursing Corps Museum (QARANC) holds a number of collections of personal papers (at QARANC Regimental HQ, Aldershot).

A few words about the papers of individuals should be said. No one involved in nursing has left such vast quantities of writings behind as Florence Nightingale, whose copious correspondence is represented in libraries in nearly every corner of the world. Some memorabilia, reminiscences, etc. relating to war service of individual nurses is located in the QARANC Museum mentioned above, and the Imperial War Museum, and a few collections in the Wellcome Institute also relate to either the First or Second World War. The memoirs of a Crimean War nurse are to be found in the Royal Army Medical Corps Muniment Collection (RAMC 532). For civil nursing there is rather less: the papers of a Director of Nursing Studies are held in the Lothian Health Board archives, and the CMAC holds a few small collections of individuals' papers, but on the whole this is an aspect of nursing history which is particularly under-represented in archive and manuscript sources.

Finally, a few words on oblique and unexpected sources for nurses and nursing. Records of related professions such as mid-wifery and health visiting may be of use: the Royal College of Midwives holds copious material on the rise of the professional-ized midwife, while the archives of the Health Visitors' Associ-ation, and of the Chartered Society of Physiotherapy, are both held in the CMAC at the Wellcome Institute. Records of medical organizations, such as the British Medical Association, contain material on professional relations, perhaps predictably. The papers of Marie Stopes, both those at the Wellcome Institute and those in the British Library, contain considerable material on her clinic nurses – she thought, on principle, that birth control advice ought to be given by trained nurses, who would have more rap-port with the poor women she sought to aid, rather than doctors who might intimidate them. Among the material which survives are several examination papers completed by nurses desirous of working in the clinics, and the regular reports returned by these nurses to Stopes on the work of the Clinic. The Family Planning Association archive in the CMAC also includes material on nurses in family planning work.

HOSPITAL RECORDS

Although public records, hospital records are not held by the Public Record Office, except in some few cases as an interim measure, but do have to be held in a repository which has been approved by the Lord Chancellor. In most cases this means a local authority record office, although some hospital records are in university archives and some material in local history libraries and museums. A number of hospitals still retain their own archives, with varying standards of storage and archival care. In some cases they are to be found heaped up in basement or attic, in constant danger of being thrown out as rubbish. In other cases there is an honorary archivist, someone who has been connected with the hospital for a long time and who is interested in its history, usually a retired or semi-retired consultant. While such honoraries may do valuable work in retrieving the records from all corners of the hospital, there is always the danger that when they finally depart there is no one to continue the work. A few health authorities, chiefly in London, appointed professional archivists to look after their records; however, because of continuing competition for resources, most of these posts are of somewhat precarious tenure and because of changes within the NHS, no longer directly funded by health authorities.

Too often within hospitals there is little awareness of the status of their records and from time to time there are in fact cases of records being found in skips, on rubbish tips, or – more positively – saved from the bonfire. Strayed volumes even turn up in private hands. A few years ago my colleague Julia Sheppard and I contacted *The Lancet* following an article in which a doctor mentioned possessing a 'leather-bound ledger' from a hospital he had once worked at, and it is pleasing to relate that this volume is now reunited at the Greater London Record Office with the series from which it had strayed. While in some cases individuals save records from near-certain destruction this is only a stay of execution if these volumes remain in their attic and get thrown out when the house is cleared.

At the Contemporary Medical Archives Centre a database on hospital records in approved repositories is maintained jointly with the Public Record Office. One of the fields under which records are classified and can be searched on is nursing records. Other fields which can be used for searching are: status of hospital (voluntary, poor law, local authority or private [pre-1948], NHS, trust, or private [post-1948]), type of hospital (general, isolation, mental, maternity, tuberculosis, women and children and other [pre-1948], acute, geriatric, maternity, mental/psychiatric and other [post-1948]), and specific town or county. It is also possible to search under hospital name to see if records of a particular type survive.

A search has thrown up 255 hospitals out of 1,812 on the database for which records specifically of nursing survive, covering a wide range of institutions: voluntary hospitals, teaching hospitals, poor law infirmaries, cottage hospitals, mental hospitals, children's hospitals (including some with further specialization, e.g. hip disease or heart trouble), maternity hospitals, hospitals for

women, isolation hospitals, the Seamen's Hospital, the Elizabeth
Garrett Anderson Hospital, cancer and other specialist hospitals,
in a wide variety of locations in England, Wales and Scotland.
There are therefore surviving records for nursing in a wide variety
of types of institution and specialities. In addition a manual register is kept of material gleaned otherwise than by the deliberate
circulation of repositories, which does not as yet fit readily into
the format of the database which is, however, constantly being
updated, and we hope will eventually incorporate this less structured information.

The database is not only a valuable tool for the researcher in
locating material, it also provides a basis on which archivists can
make decisions when faced with the very large amounts of
material generated by hospitals over the past century or so, as it
is possible to find out what already survives in what areas of the
country. While we should all like to preserve as much as possible,
limited resources mean decisions have to be taken as to what to
keep and what not to keep and the information in the hospital
records database shows both gaps, where possibly further efforts
should be made to locate and preserve material, and areas which
are already rich in surviving archival material, thus providing a
basis for the establishment of priorities.

It is hoped that the data will, in the not too distant future, be
transferred into a more user-friendly database package, which
could then be made available to users at terminals within the
Wellcome Institute Library and at the Public Record Office, and,
like the Library catalogues, via JANET (Joint Academic
Network). However, at the moment CMAC staff will undertake
simple searches for enquirers, either by name of hospital, or a
first sift for specific types of records, for example, nursing records
of tuberculosis hospitals between 1900 and 1950. If further consultation needs to be undertaken beyond that level the researcher
would be expected to make an appointment to come to the
Wellcome Institute and use the database under the supervision
of a member of staff.

Hospital records became public records as a result of the inception of the National Health Service: there has been considerable
anxiety lately about the status of hospital archives with the
changes taking place within the NHS and, as at August 1996, no
definitive statement on this subject seems to have appeared. A
Department of Health circular, HC(89)20, 'Health Services Man-

agement: Preservation, Retention, and Destruction of Records: Responsibilities of Health Authorities under the Public Records Acts' was issued in 1989. It is now being looked at for further revision, but given the time it took to revise the earlier circular of 1961 (HM (61)73) in the light of over twenty years of considerable changes in local government and the health service (and increasing interest in medical history), there seems little ground for optimism that anything will appear in the immediate future. The rather misleadingly named Health Authorities Archivists Group (formed in the late 1980s as a forum for archivists employed within hospital archives or with a particular interest in this area) is monitoring the situation and is producing its own guidelines to the selection of clinical records.

DANGERS TO ARCHIVES, AND WHAT TO DO ABOUT THEM

Archives are in constant danger: from wear and tear, inadequate storage, moves and administrative changes. What can be done? One thing is to be aware that organizations and individuals may hold papers which are of no current interest but may be of great historical significance. Within organizations, the establishment of good records management practice ensures that current and non-current files never reach that overwhelming stage at which the only solution seems to be to throw everything out to free the space. Once material has been designated as archival, decisions have then to be made about what to do with it. Does the organization want to retain it? Members of the organization should be aware of the ways to minimize physical damage to documents and the means of extending their life through good storage and handling. Ideally, if organizations are making their archives available to researchers, this should be under supervision for good security – admittedly a counsel of perfection.

And these are only the problems of institutions or individuals with a settled home. The dangers facing the records of organizations which have no permanent home, and a circulating secretariat, are even greater, as in the case of the records of the Association of Health and Residential Care Officers, formerly the National Association of Masters and Matrons of Poor Law Institutions (now in the Contemporary Medical Archives Centre). This body was founded in 1898 but minutes only survive from

1915, with a large gap from 1933 to 1946. The official library of yearbooks and publications still extant in 1964 was no longer with the archive in 1985; a clearing out of files took place in 1969. Secretarial correspondence goes back to the mid-1950s, and there are some files on important constitutional matters from the 1940s, but apart from these, and the minutes, hardly anything survives prior to 1960.

It may well be decided by an organization, or indeed an individual, that in order to liberate space for current activities, and to make the material more readily accessible to the researcher, or, of course, to ensure that the non-current records are preserved at all, the archives should be placed in some appropriate repository. Nearly all counties in England and Wales have a county record office, and a number of cities also have record offices, while a glance through *British Archives* will indicate what very various and specialized repositories exist.[13] Some records (e.g. those of hospitals) are legally public records and the Public Record Office Liaison Officer should be consulted, to advise on approved places of deposit. The British Records Association Records Preservation Section also advises on these questions. In most cases the local record office will be the appropriate repository, although in the case of nursing records a professionally run hospital archive may be the right place, and in some cases the local university may be interested, particularly if nurse education now falls within their purlieu. The Contemporary Medical Archives Centre at the Wellcome Institute is always willing to advise and in some cases might be the appropriate place of deposit. The CMAC is also prepared to undertake brief on-site surveys of archives within the immediate vicinity of London, in order to advise on care and preservation.

It can thus be seen that in spite of the difficulties mentioned in tracing nurses in the archives, and though there are many areas for which little documentation exists, there does in fact exist a great deal of material, very little of which has yet been much explored by historians.

SOME USEFUL ADDRESSES

British Records Association (Records Preservation Section), 18 Padbury Court, London EC2 7EH
Contemporary Medical Archives Centre, Wellcome Institute for the

History of Medicine, 183 Euston Road, London NW1 2BE. Tel: 0171
611 8483/2/5 Fax: 0171 611 8703.
Greater London Record Office, 40 Northampton Road, London EC1R
0HB
Health Authorities Archivists' Group, c/o Andrew Griffin, Archivist,
City and Hackney Health Authority, St Bartholomew's Hospital, West
Smithfield, London EC1A 7BE
National Register of Archives, Quality House, Quality Court, Chancery
Lane, London WC2 1HP
Public Record Office, Ruskin Avenue, Kew, Surrey TW9 4DU
Royal College of Nursing (Archivist), 42 South Oswald Road, Edinburgh
EH9 2HH

NOTES

1 J. Foster and J. Sheppard, 'Archives and the History of Nursing', in
  C. Davies (ed.), *Rewriting Nursing History*, London, Croom Helm,
  1980.
2 Ibid.
3 F. Nightingale, *Notes on Nursing: What it is and What it is not*,
  London, Harrison (1860). See also manuals of domestic management
  from the seventeenth to the mid-twentieth century for the assumption
  that nursing the sick was an integral part of the duties of a woman
  running a household.
4 R. White, *Social Change and the Development of the Nursing Profession: A Study of the Poor Law Nursing Service, 1848–1948*, London,
  Henry Kimpton, 1978.
5 Personal communication from Dr Anne Summers.
6 B. Abel-Smith, *A History of the Nursing Profession*, London, Heinemann, 1960, p. 10.
7 Minutes of the Elizabeth Fry Protestant Nursing Sisters, December
  1941, archives of the Queen's Nursing Institute in the Contemporary
  Medical Archives Centre, Wellcome Institute for the History of Medicine: cataloguing in progress.
8 'Register of Nurses', records of the Elizabeth Fry Protestant Nursing
  Sisters among the archives of the Queen's Nursing Institute in the
  Contemporary Medical Archives Centre, Wellcome Institute for the
  History of Medicine: cataloguing in progress.
9 J. Moore, *A Zeal for Responsibility: The Struggle for Professional
  Nursing in Victorian England, 1868–1883*, Athens, GA and London,
  University of Georgia Press, 1988, has used archives in the Greater
  London Record Office (St John's House eventually amalgamated
  with St Thomas's Hospital and its records are among its archives
  there), King's College Library, and in the Birmingham mother-house
  of the Nursing Sisters of St John the Divine.
10 Ibid.
11 A. Summers, *Angels and Citizens: British Women as Military Nurses,
   1854 to 1914*, London, Routledge & Kegan Paul, 1988.

12 S. McGann, 'The Archives of the Royal College of Nursing', *History of Nursing Society Journal*, 1992, vol. 4, no. 3, pp. 117–24.
13 J. Foster and J. Sheppard, *British Archives: A Guide to Archive Resources in the United Kingdom: 3rd edn.*, London, Macmillan, 1995.

Index

Page numbers in bold denote major section/chapter devoted to subject